D0044435

PRAISE FOR
Pleasurable Weight Loss

"How can weight loss be pleasurable? You've got to be kidding, right? No—not kidding. In fact, the entire solution to sustainable body confidence and permanent weight loss is pleasure. And this book outlines the path. Delightfully."

CHRISTIANE NORTHRUP, MD
Bestselling author of *Women's Bodies, Women's Wisdom* and *The Wisdom of Menopause*

"Women are hungry for creative new approaches to weight loss. Through ten years of coaching, Jena la Flamme has devised a unique and pleasurable approach to a topic often filled with pain and suffering."

JOSHUA ROSENTHAL
Founder of Institute for Integrative Nutrition and author of *Integrative Nutrition: Feed Your Hunger for Health and Happiness*

"Jena la Flamme is at the leading edge of a new era in weight loss for women. She takes a powerful stand for us to enjoy food, enjoy our bodies to become healthy and vibrantly alive in the process. If you want to enjoy the skin you're in and get the body you've always wanted, look no further. Jena will guide you every pleasurable step of the way."

MARIE FORLEO
Creator of Marie TV

"*Pleasurable Weight Loss* not only offers a path for weight loss from a gifted weight-loss coach—in the process of coaching us on weight loss, she is a brilliant activator of joy, well-being, and—above all—pleasure. She is an original genius at transforming this challenging subject into a new way of life for us all. I highly recommend it."

BARBARA MARX HUBBARD
Founder of Foundation for Conscious Evolution

"Jena's brilliant approach to weight loss is as powerful as it is practical. It tosses aside the ideas of shame, diet, and deprivation and instead embraces a more gentle, sympathetic, and loving relationship between yourself and your body. I recommend her teachings and her approach to many of my clients, as she delivers excellent results."

JON GABRIEL
Bestselling author of *The Gabriel Method: The Revolutionary Diet-Free Way to Totally Transform Your Body*

"Jena la Flamme offers a practical and sexy path to transform our relationship to food, to reclaim trust in our cravings, to connect to the love within us, and to remember that our body is our sacred chance to be here."
MEGGAN WATTERSON
Author of *REVEAL: A Sacred Manual For Getting Spiritually Naked*

"*Pleasurable Weight Loss* is revolutionary and this book will inspire you to give yourself exactly what you need to have the body and life you want."
ALEXANDRA JAMIESON
Gourmet healthy chef and author of *The Great American Detox Diet*

"Jena teaches women that there's no reason to wait until you're thin to start feeling happy or sexy. In this book, she shows you how connecting with what makes you happy is the secret to losing weight and keeping it off. I couldn't agree more."
MARCI SHIMOFF
Bestselling author of *Happy for No Reason*

"Hormone balance is the key to sustainable weight loss and in this revolutionary book, Jena la Flamme shows us how inviting pleasure into our lives—and freeing ourselves from the guilt we've been conditioned to associate with pleasure—is the recipe to recreate hormonal balance. Read this book. Your body will thank you."
SARA GOTTFRIED, MD
Bestselling author of *The Hormone Cure*

"This book rocked my world! I received an absolutely critical piece in the body/mind/spirit puzzle from this book that had previously been missing and I'm so grateful."
KATE NORTHRUP
Author of *Money: A Love Story*

"Never before has anyone made losing weight more enjoyable! Jena offers fun, simple-to-understand advice that makes reaching your goals exciting and attainable. She truly helps you build the self-esteem you need in order to fully love yourself and to achieve real, lasting results!"
CYNTHIA PASQUELLA, CCN
Author of *PINK Method* and *Hungry Hottie Cookbook*

"Jena la Flamme has exquisitely woven a clear path back into yourself and into your own radiant beauty by inviting you to reclaim your birthright of pleasure. Brilliant book, a must read for all women."

SAIDA DÉSILETS, PHD
Author of *The Emergence of the Sensual Woman*

"I lost 40 pounds applying Jena's approach, which is step-by-step oriented and concrete, yet invites self-exploration and subtle changes. I've found that the more I am able to exercise my femininity, the more the overeating has just fallen away. I realized that my weight gain wasn't about a lack of will power (as most other diets would say) and it wasn't about a lack of self-control. It was about me filling a void inside of myself. When I was able to fill that void with other ways that were so much more nourishing than a bag of potato chips, I didn't need to overeat to keep myself afloat."

SARAH JENKS
Founder of Live More Weigh Less

"This book is a life-changer! Once you've discovered her holistic approach to pleasurable weight loss, you'll never go back!"

ROSE COLE
Transformational guide and author of *High Priestess Training*

"This is a wonderful book and a game-changing read for anyone who struggles with her weight . . . full of great concepts and tips and written in a simple, approachable way. Jena shows us that by feeling good on the inside, we can make beautiful changes on the outside. This is a deeply refreshing and important book that can change your body and your life—in the most pleasurable way possible."

RENEE STEPHENS
Author of *Full-Filled: The 6 Week Weight-Loss Plan for Changing Your Relationship with Food—and Your Life—from the Inside Out*

"Jena is a gifted teacher who speaks from her own personal vulnerability and truth. With her power to tap inside a woman's inner world, Jena will guide you to awaken the power inside of you to show you the way to freedom. Through Jena's work, not only will women lose weight, they will also release years (or a lifetime) of shame."

ANDRÉA ALBRIGHT
Author of *Thin in 30 Minutes*

"It's refreshing to hear a perspective on eating that revolves around giving ourselves what we really need—enjoyment, aliveness, connection—rather than focusing on what we already have too much of in our life—restraint, control, and denial. Jena shows us that when connected to pleasure, your relationships with your body, food, and weight all become easy." ISABEL FOXEN DUKE
Emotional eating expert and creator of Stop Fighting Food

"I used to feel guilty about feeling too good in my body, which had me hold onto weight—no matter how much I exercised or dieted. After reading Jena's book and applying her work in my life, I feel the best I ever have in my body, while eating exactly as I love to, and moving my body with joy and love."
ALEXIS NEELY
Author and founder of Eyes Wide Open Life
and New Law Business Model

"When a woman steps fully into her pleasure, she is freed to be the power that she is—this is a radical act of love. Jena la Flamme invites us into this freedom, this love, so that we can be fully here now. Follow her undulating steps to remember the divine, passionate, pleasurable woman you are."
ELAYNE KALILA DOUGHTY, MA, MFT

"Jena la Flamme's work is turning the entire weight loss industry on its head. Her ideas are truly revolutionary, and they work. Yes, women lose weight, but they gain so much more. Her work guides women into true, radical love of themselves, their bodies, and their lives. I know—I am one of those women. I am so excited for every woman who gets her hands on this book. Her life will—joyfully—never be the same." KC BAKER
Founder of The Women's Thought Leadership Society

PLEASURABLE WEIGHT LOSS

PLEASURABLE WEIGHT LOSS

THE SECRETS TO FEELING GREAT,
LOSING WEIGHT,
AND LOVING YOUR LIFE TODAY

jena la flamme

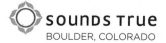
sounds true
BOULDER, COLORADO

Sounds True
Boulder, CO 80306

Published 2015

Book design by Rachael Murray

The passage printed on pages 73–74 is from the book *A Return to Love*
by Marianne Williamson. Copyright © 1992 by Marianne Williamson.
Reprinted by permission of HarperCollins Publishers.

Printed in the United States of America

Library of Congress Cataloging-in-Publication Data
  La Flamme, Jena.
  Pleasurable weight loss : the secrets to feeling great, losing weight,
  and loving your life today / Jena la Flamme.
     pages cm
  Includes bibliographical references and index.
  ISBN 978-1-62203-414-7 (alk. paper)
  1. Weight loss—Psychological aspects. 2. Overweight women—Psychology.
  3. Pleasure—Psychological aspects. I. Title.
  RM222.2.L252 2014
  613.2'5—dc23
                                        2014030487

Ebook ISBN 978-1-62203-450-5

10 9 8 7 6 5 4 3 2 1

FOR MICHAEL ELLSBERG
This book will always be our baby

RECEIVE FREE ARTICLES, VIDEOS, INVITATIONS
to Complimentary Classes, and Bonus Content
Exclusive to this Book—Join My Email List

As a thank you for buying this book, I would like to email you two companion bonuses, *The Secrets of Pleasurable Style Guide* and *Guided Meditations*. To access them for free, go to PleasurableWeightLoss.com/secretbonus and enter your email address. When you join my list you'll also receive articles, video content, and invitations to my webinars and free online classes.

The Secrets of Pleasurable Style Guide will show you how to have more pleasure in your life immediately by learning how to dress for your shape. Simply dressing in a way that flatters your body can make you look ten pounds lighter in an instant. Discover your personal style, the wardrobe essentials every woman needs to feel great in her body, and many other secrets of pleasurable style.

Guided Meditations will help you integrate the teachings in this book with your daily life. They have been developed to help you shift your relationships with your female body, eating, and pleasure. This exclusive audio content can be downloaded so that you can take the meditations with you wherever you go.

I send only quality content to my email list—no spam—and I will never give your information to anyone else. You can remove yourself at any time with one click. Enjoy these gifts with my gratitude.

Contents

foreword
By Mama Gena

THERE ARE MOMENTS of unasked for, unexpected grace that can occasionally happen in the lifetime of an educator. One of those moments is encountering a student who is so filled with passion, joy, and enthusiasm for the work that she gives even more than she receives from the class she is taking. The other moment is when a student takes the material and carves her own magnificent trail in the world, taking herself and everyone in her pathway higher because of her voice and her deepest soul's calling. Jena la Flamme has given me both gifts, and more. With this extraordinary book, I have had the remarkable experience of witnessing my dear friend Jena step into her voice as a leader in the Pleasure Revolution and as a leader for women in the world. And I had the privilege of learning so much, personally, from her incredible research and creativity in the world of women, pleasure, and weight loss.

Whether we are fat or thin, young or old, every woman I have ever encountered struggles, not only with weight, but as Jena so brilliantly points out, with every aspect of her relationship with her body. We don't trust our own intuition, we don't treat ourselves with reverence, we ignore our deepest truths and deepest longings, and we devalue the importance of pleasure. Looking for what's wrong with ourselves is so deeply ingrained; we can't even sense what's right. It has taken thousands of years of a patriarchal culture to teach women to hate themselves, doubt themselves, and mistrust themselves to the degree that we do. In this incredibly powerful book, Jena gracefully and gently leads us to a whole new world of love and partnership with the most important people in our lives—ourselves. Essentially, she undoes a millennium of negativity in a single well-crafted volume.

I have been teaching women about pleasure for over twenty years, and Jena opened my heart, mind, and body to a whole new paradigm. When she described her revelation, in the very first chapter, that her body was a perfect female animal who knew everything it needed to know, who knew every way it needed to move, who she could trust to know everything it needed to eat and every pleasure it required to fill its soul, I was stopped in my tracks. I had never ever thought of my body in that way, and I could hear my female animal not just sigh with relief, but enthusiastically take me by the hand as if to show me, teach me, and tell me everything she had wanted me to know and hear and benefit from. For years, my own female animal had been longing to collaborate with me and guide me, but I had not ever trusted her enough to pay attention. It was the greatest gift to finally reconnect with myself in a way I had never even dreamed possible. To find out that *I* was my own best ally has been such a game changer for me. Not only have I lost weight, but I am actually enjoying the fun of collaborating with myself. Each day, each meal has turned from a struggle of disapproval, restriction, and guilt to an interesting dialogue of desire and enjoyment. In fact, now that I have turned over the controls to my beautiful female body, my desire to binge on carbs or indulge in way too much chocolate has disappeared. I can *feel* myself, and I can feel how the food impacts my well-being. Instead of making a decision to overeat because I am emotionally wrought or feeling deprived, my new deal with my body is that she can have anything she wants, anything that will bring her pleasure, anything that she desires. Therefore, I actually find I want to choose things that will make me feel great, and I no longer operate from a sense of deprivation. Wow. This is a whole new world of experience for me, where every day becomes an adventure in pleasure rather than an adventure in restriction and distortion.

Jena not only brilliantly navigates a woman's relationship with food, but also applies her genius to movement and exercise. What woman wouldn't want to learn to move in a way that is natively *woman?* Jena opens her readers' imaginations to try forms of exercise and movement that are innately feminine, enabling us to connect even more deeply to our beautiful female animals. After reading about Jena's adventures with salsa, I cannot wait to try it myself.

I am so excited for every woman to experience Jena's work. When women are free from shame, free from doubt, free from self-hatred, we become bold and powerful. When we stand in rapport with our bodies, we are unafraid to speak our truths, stand for our deepest beliefs, and risk the joy and vulnerability of true sisterhood.

This book is not just about pleasurable weight loss—it is a book about deepening our connection with the fun and privilege of being a woman. It's a book about connecting with our bodies in a way we have always longed for. It's a book about learning how to reconnect with our deepest intuitions and live from that sacred spot. Jena reminds all of us to be on a first-name basis with the ecstatic joy and pleasure that is possible in each and every moment. And for that, I am deeply grateful.

Regena Thomashauer (a.k.a. "Mama Gena")
New York City
January 2015

introduction
The Feminine Power of Pleasure

WELCOME, WOMAN. You're embarking on a journey that will unite you with a feminine force that will transform your body and your life—pleasure. When a woman finds her pleasure, she glows. She radiates confidence. She becomes wildly attractive. And best of all, she feels absolutely fabulous in her skin—fully relaxed yet ready to take on any challenge, including weight loss.

Over the past twelve years, I've found that the secret to losing weight is not about enjoying less but about enjoying more. I've discovered that the path to losing weight is much more than a 30-day plan: it's a whole new way of living and relating to food and your body. My techniques affect women on a deep and meaningful level, and, dare I say, with these feminine strategies, you will actually enjoy the process of losing weight.

While this is not per se a "diet" book, by following my program, you'll see weight loss results, just like the thousands of women who've worked with me. But to get the most out of the experience, you'll need to adopt a whole new perspective on weight loss. My approach is effective only when you learn to trust your female body and pleasure. The tools I share will put you on the path to profound self-love. The journey may challenge you, but I guarantee that the pursuit of feeling good in your skin is worth the effort. And when you're on the other side, you'll feel better than ever about yourself and your appearance. Surprisingly, you can accomplish all this without denying yourself the foods, or any form of pleasure, you love.

These days I trust that my body knows exactly what to eat to stay in great shape. But it wasn't always this way. I didn't always trust my body or feel beautiful. In fact, I remember clearly the first time I uttered the loaded words that ruin lives: "I'm fat."

HOW I BROKE OUT OF FOOD JAIL

I was twelve years old when I first said those words out loud, pinching the flesh at the front of my belly to prove I was correct. Yet I wasn't fat. I was a healthy girl, attending primary school in Australia and experiencing the first signs of becoming a woman. But my view of what a woman's body should look like had already been distorted by the dominant paradigm.

As I got older, I tried to lose weight by controlling my food, but I soon found that restriction had the opposite effect. My body simply could not be denied. The more I tried to control what I ate, the more I spiraled into out-of-control eating. I had a pattern of binging at breakfast and then starving myself the rest of the day, denying my appetite with the cruel indifference of a slave driver. By late afternoon, I couldn't maintain the control and would binge again, usually on foods loaded with sugar. After a binge, I would feel physically sick and emotionally overwhelmed by guilt and disgust. My imbalanced eating habits and the lack of nutritious foods brought on constipation, fatigue, and depression. Filled with shame and self-loathing, I was yet another intelligent young woman blindly caught in the grips of compulsive eating and a bad body image. And the more I failed in my attempts to lose weight, the more my upside-down opinion that my body was fundamentally flawed was reinforced. The only way I knew to make myself feel better was to eat. I was stuck in my own miserable food jail.

Then I met a man who profoundly changed my life. His name was Gum, like Australia's signature tree, the gum tree.

Gum invited me to visit him in the subtropical rainforest where he lived (and still does to this day) in a solar-powered house made of recycled materials. On the border of a World Heritage National Park, his house was nestled in a small clearing, surrounded by palms, ferns, and magnificent tall trees with thick vines. The air in this lush environment was refreshing, cool, and moist. Every imaginable shade of green was present. Back in the 1970s, Gum had been an environmental activist. His participation in direct-action protests helped to keep loggers out of the rainforest. As a result, within a few minutes' walk from his house, two- and three-thousand-year-old trees were still standing, proud and regal, supporting a vast ecology. I soon found that when I was in nature, I felt like a completely different person. I was relaxed, grounded, and more alive.

I had always been a city girl, though I'd been on many hiking trails and loved the beach and the ocean. But I was scared of the wild forest. Inside Gum's house, I knew I was safe; the surrounding wilderness, however, remained a frightening unknown. Eager to initiate me to the ways of nature, Gum took me on off-trail hikes deep into the wilderness. As he showed me how to be in harmony with the environment, my fear of nature began to fall away. I found that instead of being a potentially dangerous threat, Mother Nature was a kind and gentle protective force that cradled me. I built up the courage to walk into the forest alone, and I would sit in silence by the roots of a tree, observing the quietude of nature.

One day I had an experience that changed my life. I had been raised to believe that people are superior to nature and that the earth is ours to use as we please. But in a moment, while sitting in the moist mulch, feeling comfortable and safe, I felt my separation from nature melt away. In an instant, my arrogance was humbled. I realized that my body *is* nature. I was awed by the oneness I felt with every other creature and organism on the planet. I was, like them, a child of Mother Earth.

I remember sitting on the forest floor, enraptured by the glory of the ecosystem around me, when I noticed a small tree. The other trees loomed above my head, but this one was small enough for me to touch its leaves. Some had insect bites and holes or were stained with mold; others were cracked or half dead. The tree as a whole was inarguably beautiful, but its leaves were clearly imperfect. That was the first time that my fierce negative body image began to soften. It occurred to me that it might be okay for my body not to be the perfect body of magazine standards. Over time, I would return to that memory of sitting in the forest and wondering, *If this tree is beautiful in all its imperfections, why can't I be too?*

Even after these epiphanies, though, I still felt shackled by my food compulsions. I thought I knew what I was supposed to be doing to lose weight—eat less, exercise more—but I wasn't motivated to stick with any program. This is the same dilemma that millions of women face every day. In this information age, with an abundance of nutritional guidance available at the click of a mouse, why can't we simply do what we learn is best for us? The reason is simple: dieting isn't fun. It doesn't make us happy, and it certainly isn't pleasurable.

Years later, after an exhaustive search into the workings of the body and the mind, I finally found the answer I was looking for. The cure was a juicy secret: pleasure. I became a devoted disciple of pleasure. By that I don't mean blindly indulging in an ice cream fantasy, although there is a place for ice cream in my life. What I learned was that to lose weight, I needed to let go of my old beliefs about pleasure, adopt a new way of looking at my body, and embrace a few easy methods to experience a new sense of pleasure—whenever I desire. I learned to recognize when a nonedible source of joy would soothe my soul more than another glass of chardonnay or another helping of pasta. And I was finally able not only to enjoy each bite of delicious food but also to recognize when I'd had enough. The implications of choosing pleasure rippled into other areas of my life, too, which became richer and more fulfilling.

Contrary to what you might think, pleasure is not childish or frivolous. It requires perspective, maturity, and wisdom. The Greek philosopher Epicurus, from whose name and philosophy the term *epicurean delight* derives, wrote, "It is impossible to live pleasurably without living wisely, well, and justly. And it is impossible to live wisely, well, and justly without living pleasurably."

Clearly, pleasure's reputation has been dragged through the mud. It is misunderstood to be a shallow enterprise rather than the path of wisdom it actually is.

One of the most widely circulated myths about pleasure is that it is a lazy and passive approach to life. Nothing could be further from the truth! The lazy way to go about life is to follow the path laid out by society's expectations. When you surrender to the tow of the dominant paradigm, trust me, you will not experience true pleasure. Laziness will lead you down a path of averageness, with average relationships, average work, and an average life, which these days will mean averagely depressed or anxious, averagely overweight, and averagely hating your body. Pleasure, on the other hand, calls for something completely different. As Regena Thomashauer (a.k.a. "Mama Gena") writes, "Pleasure is the highest form of responsibility."

I had always perceived pleasure as something that happens to you, if you're lucky, through outside forces. But I was missing the point—my hands control the pleasure dial of my life. Once I understood this, I broke free from the bondage of emotional eating, weight struggles, and a bad body image. Not only did I escape food jail, but I tore down its walls and danced on their ruins. The lessons I learned became my life's work. Today, I teach women across the globe how to escape from the same misery and instead live their lives enjoying food and reveling in their bodies.

When we create a life that is truly pleasurable, our relationship with food becomes more natural and intuitive, and when we learn to eat with pleasure, the brain and the body work together to tell us when to eat and when to stop, without the need for restriction or control. These are not woo-woo New Age concepts; they are supported by the latest science on brain function, metabolism, and digestion.

I now have the body, the body image, and the relationship with food I always wished for, and I have been able to maintain all three for more than ten years. I enjoy food without reservation, without restriction, and without having to worry about my weight. I've seen amazing transformations occur when pleasure is fully embraced as a part of life—first with myself and then with thousands of my clients. Now it's your turn.

THE PLEASURABLE WEIGHT LOSS APPROACH

My method will allow you to experience your body in a whole new way that will delight your soul. You will discover what your body loves and what it doesn't, not only with food but also with your sensuality, sexuality, physical movement, friendships, and more. When you follow the Pleasurable Weight Loss approach you'll see that there are no food rules, regulations, points, or calorie counting. I'll show you not only how to actually enjoy yourself on your weight loss journey but also how enjoying food and life are essential—without accessing pleasure, you'll never succeed.

The Pleasurable Weight Loss approach is a softer, more graceful way to achieve weight loss, and you will be happy to know that it works. You'll learn to trust and work with the wisdom of your body rather than fight against it. The truth is that your beautiful body already knows what to eat and how to move to be in its best shape, but it can't be its best when it's chronically stressed. Pleasure is the trigger that moves the body away from stress and toward relaxation. When we're relaxed, we're able not only to let go of fears and shame surrounding our bodies but also to experience the metabolic benefits of relaxation. The body burns calories more effectively when it is relaxed.

Come with me to explore your deepest desires. They will be the catalyst for a relaxed state of mind that will help you lose weight, ramping up your metabolism without any additional effort. Your desires will guide you through a multifaceted experience of pleasurable weight loss and more.

- **Embrace the wisdom of your female animal.**
  Instead of looking outside yourself by following yet another diet, you can learn how to listen to the voice of your female body. Like all animals in nature, she already knows how to eat and move to be in balance. You will hear her when you are in a relaxed state. Your female animal is stronger than your rational mind, which is why in order to heal your relationship with food and lose weight sustainably, you must embrace her feminine wisdom.

- **Embody the science of pleasurable weight loss.** Science shows that stress can cause weight gain. Fortunately, the reverse is also true: relaxation, pleasure, and sensuality create the metabolic conditions that stimulate weight loss. Pleasure is a trustworthy, intelligent guiding force. It is a vital daily nutrient. Instead of controlling, restricting, and pushing yourself, you'll learn to awaken your senses to pleasure, so that you can feel more, savor more, and enjoy this feminine approach to weight loss.

- **Create your ideal ecology for pleasurable weight loss.** Animals thrive in the right natural environment. Your body can also thrive when you create its ideal ecology, which includes your external environment, as well as your thoughts and beliefs. Pleasurable weight loss will naturally occur when the right inner and outer conditions are in place.

- **When sexy is safe, you'll lose weight.** Weight gain is your body's cry for attention, and its attempt at self-protection. You may be intimidated by the attention that comes with having a sexy body, and you may think you need to lose weight to be sexy. But until you learn to "handle the heat," the many projections that society puts on a sexy woman, you may subconsciously sabotage yourself by retreating to the fridge for the safety and insulation of extra weight. I'll show you how you can begin to feel sexy just as you are now, and I'll show you how your "turn-on" will literally turn on your metabolism, heightening your body's calorie-burning efficiency to support pleasurable weight loss.

- **Nourish your animal with pleasurable eating and pleasurable cooking.** Learn how to eat with pleasure—bite by bite—enjoying anything your heart desires until you're completely satisfied, whether you're at home or at a restaurant. I have included dozens of delicious and easy-to-prepare recipes to turn your kitchen into a haven of health.

- **Enjoy pleasurable movement.** You may think you can lose weight by exercising even if you don't enjoy it. But any exercise that your body experiences as punishing actually has the opposite effect: it stimulates a stress response that causes you to gain weight, not lose it! I'll explain why pleasurable movement is the only sustainable way for you to transform your shape.

- **Implement my techniques with "Pleasure Practices" and "Pleasure Bites."** The suggestions and exercises in this book will connect you to the wisdom of your body. Many of the techniques have a physical component; others require some deep thinking. Pleasure Practices and Pleasure Bites show you how to put my teachings into action so that you can start your transformation while you read this book.

- **Discover pleasurable eating practices.** When it comes to losing weight in a pleasurable way, it's not only what you eat but also how you eat that makes the difference. Pleasurable eating practices are deceptively simple, yet they are some of the most important secrets to a balanced relationship with food and your body. These practices are central to the teachings of pleasurable weight loss.

It's now time to toss aside any ideas that treating yourself to what gives you pleasure is selfish. It's time to start afresh. This is going to be a wonderful adventure! You will finally throw away the scale, ditch the diet food, and get to know the beautiful and radiant woman you were born to be. Enjoy the ride!

To lose confidence in one's body is to lose confidence in one's self.

SIMONE DE BEAUVOIR

1 Embracing the Wisdom of Your Female Animal

YOUR FEMALE BODY is capable of amazing feats. Pleasurable weight loss is one of them. I'm here to teach you the secrets you need to know to lose weight effortlessly and to keep it off for good. It all begins with being respectful to your body—starting right now.

It's helpful to think of your body as your own personal plot of Mother Earth, tapped into the intelligence of nature, just as powerfully as any other living creature or plant. Think about it: without the mind's direction, the body's heartbeat and breath keep it alive. What's more, the female body miraculously creates, births, and nurtures the lives of whole new beings. When you are fully connected to your body's wisdom, you'll have no problem figuring out what to eat or how to move to be fit. At that point, losing weight will be second nature.

I wasn't always in tune with my body's messages, though. I struggled with compulsive eating as a teenager and throughout part of my adult life. I hated my body and felt like I was in food jail. I was caught in a punishing cycle of binging and restricting. I thought that the discipline of control was the only way to lose weight.

A day came, however, more than ten years ago, when I first heard my body's voice talk to me. I was standing on the deck of a floating barge near the banks of the Hudson River with movement educator Bill Hedberg. After hearing me drone on with tales of woe about my years of compulsive eating and body shame, Bill asked me, "Would you like to get over your struggle with food and weight?"

"Yes, of course I would," I replied. "I just don't know how."

"I know how," he said matter-of-factly. "The reason you're still struggling is you're not listening to her."

"Listening to who?" I asked.

"Your body, Jena," he replied. "Right now, you think you're the voice in your head, but that's only one part of you. In reality, there are two of you. There's your mind, and there's your body. And your body is an *animal,* specifically a female animal. Your body is a *she,* not an *it.* She's a warm-blooded, furry creature, and she is directly connected to the wisdom of nature. Your mind is intelligent, but your body is also intelligent, in different ways. All this time you've been thinking your body isn't worth listening to, but she is."

Bill paused to see how this was landing, and seeing that I was enraptured, he carried on, sharing teachings that changed my life. "All animals in nature know what to eat to be in balance, Jena. And yours is no exception. The problem is you haven't been respecting her."

All of a sudden, I felt her ears prick up on the sides of my head, as if she had just heard her name for the very first time. Her voice cried out too, "Hello! At last! Finally someone is acknowledging me. I am wise, and I do know what to eat. I'm aware of much more than you've ever been willing to give me credit for. I haven't revealed my secrets to you because you have never sincerely inquired. You've been treating me like your enemy!"

I gulped. I was guilty as charged. Suddenly, I could see all the years of pain I had inflicted upon my body with my compulsive eating and bad body image. Until this moment, I had blamed my body for my problems with food and weight. I was certain it was my body that had wronged me. I thought that the bloating, headaches, and energy crashes were my body's fault. I hadn't connected the dots to realize that the bloating, headaches, and energy crashes were reactions; they were my body's attempts to communicate the consequences of my compulsive eating.

With a new perspective, though, I could interpret my symptoms as my body's way of telling me that this was not what she wanted. When she felt bad, it meant that whatever I was eating felt bad to her. I could see now that her warnings were clear but that I had been ignoring them. Where I had previously felt she had betrayed me, I now realized it was I who had blindly betrayed her.

I had regarded my body as a possession, something I owned and could use (or abuse) as I pleased. I was now beginning to understand that my body is not a possession but rather my mind's partner—a living, breathing, feeling, and wise female animal that belongs to life itself. The blame I'd projected onto my body for years flashed before my eyes. Now, I was rapidly becoming aware that my body was not the culprit. I realized that my body *is* smarter than I had been willing to consider. There were the times I had tripped but caught myself before hitting the ground, or the times when I'd had a cut and the wound healed. It wasn't my mind that was in charge then—it was my body! Once I recognized how brilliant my body is, my anger and resentment toward her began to melt away. For the very first time, instead of focusing on complaints about my body's appearance, I began to bask in wonder and awe at all she does for me.

I knew then that to lose weight and to find peace with food and my body I had to start listening to my female animal. As soon as I began to own the damage I had inflicted upon my body with my crude treatment, as soon as I restored to her a sense of dignity, my body responded. I felt a surge of energy well up inside of me. And that was the moment, for the first time, when I fully felt her. My body. My female animal.

I had been treating my body as if she owed me something, but the truth was very different: it was I who owed her for my participation in life. I became painfully aware that when the body dies, the life we know ends. In that respect, your body, your female animal, is your very access to life.

I also began to see my pattern of putting my attention on only her flaws. I remembered all the cruel words I'd used to describe her: disgusting, gross, fat, and worse. For the first time, I realized how much it hurt her to hear me talk about her like that. I had been so preoccupied with my mind's righteous criticism of my body that I never noticed how much anguish and stress it gave her to be accused in this way.

This was when the whole game changed for me, and the seeds of the Pleasurable Weight Loss approach were laid. Once I stopped trying to control my body and instead started listening to her, a paradigm shift occurred. As my view of my body shifted from *it,* a possession of my mind, to *she,* a living creature, my entire notion of what my "problem" was also changed. As these realizations sank in, I was also filled with an enormous sense of gratitude for my body—a 180-degree shift. My body was no longer the bane of my existence—an overweight, pain-in-the-neck source of shame. My body was now my life's heroine.

PLEASURE PRACTICE
Getting in Touch with Your Female Animal

I used to think of my body as an object that my mind could manipulate to create the body shape I wanted, but I discovered that she is a being unto herself, with wisdom to contribute to the conversation on my well-being. The concept of controlling her went out the window, and the new goal of collaborating with her took its place. How could I get along with her? How could I be in sync with her? How could I understand her needs? How could she, the body, and I, the mind, join forces? The following daily practice allows us to get back in touch with our female animals so that we can fully inhabit our bodies. Do this practice each morning and at any other time in the day when you want to connect with your animal.

Sit in a comfortable position. Take a few deep breaths to relax, right down into your lower belly. Put one hand on your belly and the other on your heart, and as you feel the breath moving in and out, sense the life force inside your body. Notice the part of you that is doing the breathing. This is your animal. She is the sensing part of you, the feeling part of you, and the female part of you. Once you wake up to her voice, you will always be able to hear her, even if at first it is only a faint whisper.

Allow your mind to relax and invite a sense of trust in the wisdom of your female body to be present. Then ask her the following questions:

- Beloved animal, what do you need right now?
- Beloved animal, what can I do to support you today?
- Beloved animal, what do you most desire?

Listen for the answers. They may be expressed as feelings, sensations, and intuitions. You might want to write them down in a journal and keep track of them. The more you listen for the voice of your female animal, the clearer it will become. Over time, you'll find it easier to discern the source of your food cravings, whether they stem from habit or your female animal. Listening to what she wants fosters better food choices, which become easier and easier.

PLEASURE BITE

Intimately connect with your animal by getting down on all fours. Feel your paws on the earth. Arch and curl your spine, and imagine you are a jungle cat with sharp instincts. Crawl, pounce, stretch, and roll on your back. Stick out your tongue and let yourself roar.

YOUR BASIC INSTINCT

All creatures in nature know how to eat to thrive. It would be absurd to think that a monkey in a tropical rainforest could be confused about what or when to eat. I began to realize that my body, like a monkey's or any other creature's body, has been groomed through the course of evolution to know how to nourish herself. She isn't stupid. Her impulses are not flawed, corrupted, or deadened, as I had feared.

Even if you've spent years abusing your female animal through compulsive, unfeeling behaviors, rest assured that her ancient wisdom cannot be lost. Over millions of years, nature has programmed your body with the wisdom to know how to nourish herself, and this instinct cannot be erased. Although your disappointing past efforts might appear to be irrefutable evidence that you should give up trying to lose weight, reinforcing a how–could–I–possibly–change–now attitude, the reality is that in Mother Nature's time frame, mere decades occur in the blink of an eye. You still have time.

Christopher Ryan, author of *Sex at Dawn: How We Mate, Why We Stray, and What It Means for Modern Relationships,* told me, "We carry the past within us. We are the past. We are designed by hundreds of thousands of years of the past that has accumulated in the shape of our bodies, in our appetites, and in the things we need to be healthy and happy. If someone thinks she can disconnect from that, then she has a very unsophisticated impression of what she is."

PLEASURE PRACTICE
The Chapel of Wonder and Awe

It's easy to fall into the trap of putting our attention on only the things we don't like about our bodies. To balance those critical voices in your head, make it a practice to notice all the brilliant things your body does for you every day. The more you notice all the ways your body supports you and allow yourself to feel gratitude for the body's wonders, the more receptive you will become to the signals she uses to communicate with you.

Let yourself feel wonder and awe for the myriad ways your body serves you every single day. You wake up every morning after a night of renewing sleep. Your feet allow you to move freely to discover the world. You digest the food that you put in your mouth. You flush out toxins and repair from a variety of illnesses and injuries. You receive pleasure through each of your senses. These are some of the many miracles your body performs in the service of keeping you alive.

Your instinct is your body's primal intuitive power. Reflect on the ways your female animal has instinctively served you well, and invoke sincere gratitude for the phenomenon of this intelligent life force.

WEIGHT LOSS IS A RELATIONSHIP ISSUE

This shift in perspective—which elevates the body from an object to a being, and in a woman's case, a feminine being—is the crux of Pleasurable Weight Loss. As soon as your body rises in status from an object without feelings to a wise female animal with guidance worthy of loving consideration, you have created a completely different dynamic for weight loss. Now that there's you and this "other," you have a relationship. Instead of weight loss being a numbers game of calories in and calories out, it becomes an intimate relationship in your life, worthy of tenderness and respect. Once you approach your body as a relationship to discover rather than a problem to fix, you start thinking in a whole new way. Embracing your instinctive female ability to nurture and applying it to the care of your female animal is the most effective strategy I've come across for losing weight in a healthy and sustainable way.

If you take a step back to look at what I'm suggesting here, you may find it ironic: I'm asking you to think about your body as a separate being in order to wake up to the need to treat her with compassion and kindness. When you think of your body as "me" or "mine," it's easy to treat her poorly. You might let your own cup run dry in a way you would never allow for others. But when you think of her as someone else, all of a sudden treating her better takes on a whole new light.

Even if you've always had a brutal relationship with food, hated how you looked, and struggled with weight for longer than you care to admit to yourself, I've seen that once a woman awakens from the cultural trance that her body is a possession or a slave of the mind, she straightaway feels drawn to treat her body more kindly. Once she grants her body the dignity of being a rightful force in her life, with whom she has a real relationship, everything changes.

A powerful tool to bring her perspective to your awareness and deepen your relationship is to continually refer to your body using the personal pronouns *she* and *her*. Do this whenever you speak of your body—most importantly, in your inner dialogue with yourself. As you've already seen, I've incorporated this practice into my life, and it has been a complete game changer.

My client Sandy once told me how this tool liberated her from the web of spinning thoughts in her sometimes confused mind. She felt so connected to the idea of using personal pronouns to describe her body that she shared the concept with her boyfriend, Richard, who enthusiastically embraced the practice. Richard thought Sandy was gorgeous, but Sandy struggled with her body image and weight. One evening, as they were thinking about what to have for dinner, Sandy started to get anxious: "I don't know what to eat! Should we go out to eat or stay home and cook?" Seeing her exasperation, Richard chimed in, "What does *she* want?"

"As soon as he said it like that, the answer came to me with crystal clarity," Sandy said. "All of a sudden, I knew that she wanted to go to our local Italian restaurant to have tilapia with potatoes and leeks, and there was no longer any confusion about it."

Understanding that weight loss is at heart a relationship is good news for women because we are hardwired to excel at relationships. We are relationship ninjas. We are daughters, sisters, mothers, aunts, and loyal friends, and we intuitively know when a relationship is healthy and when it is not. We have been programmed by evolution to ensure social harmony. We have a greater natural affinity for relationships than men, a trait that can be detected throughout every stage of our life cycle, starting as early as infancy when girls demonstrate more responsiveness than boys to the stress of others in their environment. We have a sixth sense for the unspoken needs of others, an ability related to social conditioning and a byproduct of evolution that has shaped our neural wiring.

Women are highly attuned and responsive. We can hear nuances of emotion in a voice and read the unsaid in a face. Louann Brizendine writes in *The Female Brain* that a woman's ability both to decode an infant's needs and to predict what a bigger, more aggressive male could potentially do to her gave her a distinct survival advantage.

We are not only instinctive caregivers but also proud of this trait and readily acknowledge it. We live in a culture where women are conditioned to play down our achievements—except this one. Being a great caregiver is the one thing that is culturally endorsed for a woman to have high self-esteem about, making it all the more potent a trait to hijack for pleasurable weight loss.

Once I realized that mending my relationship with my body was at the root of my challenge, what had been an obsessive quest to lose weight and heal my compulsive eating patterns took on a completely new, more inspiring quality. Where my quest had previously been all about control, it now centered on listening. Where it had been about mentally mapping "the right way" to accomplish a change, it was now about leaving room for the wordless wise guidance of my body to be heard.

Weight loss went from being a war that my mind intended to win over my body to being a team effort, an act of co-creation between two brilliant parts of myself. I knew I would never lose weight following the old rules. Once I saw the bright light of a more compassionate approach to my body, I could never turn back. From this point on, trying to lose weight without engaging my female animal and listening for her opinion seemed barbaric.

One of my personal heroes, horse whisperer Ray Hunt, had a similar transformation with his approach to horses. "I look back at how rude or crude or misunderstanding I was to the animal," says Hunt in the documentary about his work, *Turning Loose*. Hunt eventually became renowned for taming and training horses through gentleness instead of forced submission. But he didn't start out that way.

"The part that I had been overlooking was that I was working with a living, breathing, feeling, decision-making animal. I thought, if he didn't like it, too bad. I didn't think the horse was entitled to an opinion. He was just meant to do as I said," explains Hunt of his previous mindset, which mirrors the unfeeling attitude many women inflict upon their bodies in the name of weight loss.

When Hunt recognized that horses have feelings of their own, he revolutionized his training style. "It became a new challenge for me to get in harmony with the horse. To be able to do it *with* them. I wanted it to be as fun for the horse as it was going to be for me," he says in *Turning Loose*.

The partnership that you are creating between your intellect and your animal needs to be fun for both. That's why I call my approach to weight loss "pleasurable." On this journey, you'll discover how to fully enjoy this new and authentic relationship with your animal, while you relish the foods you eat and find real and lasting pleasure in all aspects of your life.

PLEASURE PRACTICE
Interviewing Your Animal

It's time to open up the lines of communication so that you can talk directly with your female animal. At first it may seem strange, as if you are talking to yourself, but soon it will be second nature to tune in to this part of yourself. Let her know of your desire to lose weight, heal your relationship with food, and enjoy your feminine body without reservation, and reassure her that you want to do it with her.

In this exercise, the mind interviews the female animal. Your mind's job is to listen intently for the voice of your animal. Your body has her unique way of speaking, and it's different from the way your mind communicates. Listen to your body and learn to be a translator.

Ask her the following questions:

- How can I make losing weight more fun for you?
- Which of your needs or desires have I been neglecting?
- What foods make you feel great?
- What makes you feel alive?
- What can I do to make you feel appreciated?
- What can I do to make you feel beautiful?

Be receptive to what you hear, and write down her answers.

LOVING YOUR ANIMAL

As you shift your experience of your body as an object and begin to animate her as a creature, she will come alive as your primary partner, particularly on your quest for pleasure. Your body is the physical part of you that allows you to experience life through the senses. Though we can enjoy the mental pleasure of a crossword puzzle or a book, the types of pleasure that are going to make the biggest difference for weight loss are those you experience through your senses.

I use many affectionate terms for my female animal, such as my girl, my lady, my partner, and my friend. And while happy, healthy, nourishing relationships with others is a crucial component of a satisfying life, the relationship you have with your body is most important. Saida Désilets, author of *Emergence of the Sensual Woman,* describes this bond between your body and mind as your "primary relationship."

You can be a rock star in all of your other relationships, but if this primary relationship between your body and mind is not flourishing, then it will cast a shadow over everything else in your life. No matter how rich you are, no matter how popular you are, and no matter how thin you are, if your primary relationship is not intimate and loving, then all other pleasures and sources of delight available to you will be soured. Losing weight offers no guarantee that you will love your body. From the stereotype of the gorgeous model who still doubts her attractiveness, to the countless women who are oblivious to how great they look and continue to be discontented with their bodies, deep down we all know, as reluctant as we may be to admit it, that it takes more than looking good to feel good about ourselves. Only when you learn to love your body unconditionally will you open the way to loving your physical form in her full feminine glory.

When you have a great primary relationship with your body, you will love your body and be in harmony with her, no matter her size. With a healthy foundation in place, when you do lose weight, you will already have practiced loving yourself unconditionally, and you will continue to do so in your new size. This understanding, that love for your body must come before lasting weight loss will occur, is one of the cornerstones of the Pleasurable Weight Loss approach.

PLEASURE BITE

Your animal desires physical attention, including the pleasure of your loving touch. Breathe deeply as you stroke your hair, caress your face, and hug your arms. Touch your breasts. Rub your belly, lower back, hips, and legs. Relish the sensations that arise.

YOUR INNER MARRIAGE

Imagine your mind and body as husband and wife, intimate partners in an inner marriage. Unlike a conventional marriage in which divorce is always an option, this body-mind marriage is truly an "until death do us part" relationship. When I began to think of my body as my faithful wife, it occurred to me that since I was "committed" to this relationship for the rest of my life, it would only make sense to give it my all to make it a good marriage. In fact, why not a great marriage? Or while I'm at it, the most passionate, delicious, loving marriage ever?

I began to ask myself two key questions: what are the qualities of an ideal marriage, and how am I going to create that relationship? Love, compassion, kindness, curiosity, creativity, passion, trust, and many other positive attributes came to mind. Above all, I thought about how ideal partners are friends. With this understanding, I was able to embrace the quest to let go of my judgment toward my body and to learn to become loving, supportive, and kind to all the different parts of me.

It should come as no surprise that cultivating this relationship requires the same level of emotional willingness you would bring to any important relationship. When I was able to disengage from my mind's critical chatter about my body, I discovered a willingness in my female animal that took my breath away. True, my body was justifiably angry at my mind for neglecting her needs. But on a deeper level, I found her to be a devoted companion who was able to forgive and forget the mistreatment of the past. She was excited to begin this relationship anew. You will find that as soon as your mind is ready to embrace your body, your female animal will be there, wagging her tail in readiness to receive your love and attention—like a puppy who greets you with warmth and enthusiasm no matter how many hours she has been left unattended.

COMPASSION: THE MAGIC INGREDIENT
OF GREAT RELATIONSHIPS

The Dalai Lama says that compassion is the radicalism of our time. To have compassion for your female animal means having sympathy for her distress and a desire to alleviate her pain. Instead of observing your body from the outside, begin sensing her experience from the inside. For example, let's say you have a craving for a cookie. It may feel as though the craving is coming from her, like she wants it and is asking for it. However, if you approach the craving with compassion and curiosity, you can climb into her universe to see what is really going on with her. Is she legitimately hungry? Is she bored? Is she angry or stressed and trying to soothe herself? Is she hungry for something unrelated to food? Allow your compassion to drive your inquiry further to consider how she will feel after she eats the cookie. Will she feel she has betrayed herself because she knows cookies don't fall in the category of the nourishing fresh foods that make her feel her best? Will she feel exhausted, helplessly succumbing to the throes of the sugar crash that follows a brief sugar high?

Compassion allows you to feel the plight of your female animal and, in doing so, puts you in touch with a new source of motivation. When you are fully aware of the impact of your actions on your female animal, you will want to meet her needs. Unlike self-pity, which may have you feeling helpless or hopeless to change, compassion opens your heart to your animal and expands your sense of possibility, restoring your power to be the creator of your own destiny.

PLEASURE PRACTICE
Providing Your Animal's Basic Needs

The basic needs of your animal are few: clean air, plenty of water, healthy food, restful sleep, daily movement, sex, shelter, companionship, relaxation, and some amount of pleasure. It has been my experience that if you are compassionate with your body and provide for her basic needs, she will be happy to cooperate with your weight loss desires. However, if the basic needs are neglected, she may stubbornly refuse to budge an ounce!

So ask yourself honestly, are you good to your animal? Are you giving her enough fresh air? Are you drinking enough water? Are you getting enough sleep? Are you connecting with quality friends? If not, these obvious foundational steps are required to lead the way to lasting pleasurable weight loss.

Next, think about your relationship with your animal. Is it an abusive relationship? A neglectful relationship? Or a kind, loving, passionate, and harmonious relationship?

Then, ask yourself: if the quality of my life and the success of my weight loss depend on my female animal being happy, what does her happiness entail? Ask your female animal, and write down your answers.

YOUR ANIMAL IS STRONG AND WISE

In *The Triune Brain in Evolution,* neuroscientist Paul MacLean explains that the human brain is made up of three distinct structures that were added sequentially during the course of evolution: the reptilian brain, the mammalian brain, and the neocortex. Each of these structures deals with a different perception of reality. The reptilian brain corresponds to the physical world; the mammalian brain, to the emotional world; and the neocortex, to the conceptual or intellectual world.

Watch a lizard in its native environment, and you'll have a good idea of what the reptilian brain is concerned with—ensuring survival and reproduction through activities such as finding food, mating, and defending its territory. The mammalian brain, also referred to as the limbic system, introduces the capacity for emotion. It is responsible for love, nurturing, and reciprocity, fostering the ability to bond with others and organize and act as a group. The neocortex provides symbolic thinking, which enables us to create narratives, invent concepts, and use language for planning and describing our perceptions.

Your female animal is governed by the combination of the reptilian and mammalian brains, which is why she often finds herself in opposition to your thinking side, or neocortex. No wonder your body cannot be held back by the willpower of your mind! With their forces combined, the reptilian and mammalian brains outnumber the neocortex two to one. So when your body reaches for one too many cookies, these more primitive parts of the brain are overriding your more advanced mind. Meanwhile, your neocortex, which wants to assert its authority, will find a reason to rationalize the action ("you worked so hard today, you deserve a few cookies"). This is why so many of us find our paws in the cookie jar day after day, even when our thinking mind knows this does not support our weight loss goals.

Let me drum this concept into you one more time. Your female animal is stronger than your highly evolved, rational mind. The conventional dieting approach fails because it tries to tame and control the untamable. Pleasurable Weight Loss succeeds because it doesn't even embark down this path of folly; instead, it seeks to cultivate the wisest possible relationship between the vastly different, but equally brilliant parts of yourself so that they can figure it out together.

RESTORING HONOR TO YOUR ANIMAL

When I joyfully share the revelation that the mind is indeed partnered with an animal, women often look at me in horror, as if I'm telling them they should be happy to be shacked up for a lifetime with an out-of-control beast! Their reaction isn't surprising. Our whole culture is based on the belief that the mind is superior to the body. The concept of original sin—wherein simply because we are conceived through sex and born through the body, we are considered sinful—is only one example that epitomizes the anti-body psychology that has been pervasive for thousands of years. Even if you were not raised religiously, do not underestimate the degree to which anti-body thinking has made its way into your mind. What may seem to you the unquestionable "truth" about your body and her worth is actually a learned belief, drilled into you since the day you were born: the body is fundamentally bad, dirty, and flawed. We get this message about all bodies, but we are taught that a woman's body is more corrupt because of its direct and symbolic association with sex.

Yet sex is one of our strongest impulses, among other needs and desires, and when we are ashamed of our bodies' natural urges or numb them out, we are effectively crippled. Women are taught not to enjoy pleasure or sex too much, and that if we do, we will be disrespected and considered a slut by the rest of society. One of my clients, who was struggling with a debilitating bad body image, grew up with a father who was a military chaplain. She asked me, "How can I learn to love my body if I hate that I am sexual?" The answer is: you can't.

When I introduce myself as a teacher of Pleasurable Weight Loss, I'm frequently asked with a muffled snicker, "You mean, this is about sex, right?" I imagine they think I make my living giving out prescriptions for "sex-ercise," and not wanting to confirm the picture in their head, I am tempted to say no. But the truest answer is yes. Pleasurable weight loss has a lot to do with sex.

Your female animal is a sexual being, born to embody her own sexual desires as well as to fulfill the desires of others. Until you can appreciate and honor your body's sexual nature and be at peace with sex, you cannot be at peace with your body—nor can you be at peace with pleasure or food. And until you are at peace with food, you will never be at peace with your weight. Therefore, discarding the shame you have about sex and pleasure is a critical leverage point for losing weight sustainably.

Although society's strongest association with sex is wrapped into shame, it hasn't always been that way. Ancient peoples didn't think sex was bad; they embraced it as powerful and magical. Archaeological evidence points to the first religious rituals as sexual rites. Early humans marveled at the role of sex in the miracle of life, which can be seen in the oldest examples of human art—rock paintings and clay figurines that depict images of female genitalia.

Pre-agricultural peoples were animists. They believed that animals, plants, and inanimate objects possessed a spiritual essence. They believed all of life was divine and honored nature. The female body was seen as a sacred vessel and a portal for life. There was a time in prehistory, before men figured out their role in conception, when women were worshipped for their presumed role as the generators of life. (I chuckle, wondering about the moment when the first woman realized the connection between her baby and the night she spent with a handsome caveman nine moons before.)

As we evolved into hunters and gatherers, we understood that we belonged to the earth, but over time, our attitude changed. We began to believe that the earth belonged to us. Earth became lesser than heaven, body lesser than mind, emotions lesser than thoughts, and women lesser than men. "Women went from being coequal, honored, central members of society to little more than breeding stock," says Christopher Ryan. With such beliefs woven into the tapestry of our culture, is it any wonder women objectify and degrade our own bodies?

That same patriarchy we have internalized is at work when we treat our bodies like possessions, with little or no regard for the body's needs. And so we employ weight loss strategies that set out to conquer our animal. Pleasurable Weight Loss is about casting off the patriarchal conditioning. It's time to truly love ourselves again. It's time to set the record straight and to restore the body to her rightful place as a trustworthy and respected guide.

Fortunately, we still have role models we can learn from as we restore this balance. Although globalization has come with devastating environmental costs, one of its blessings is the opportunity to learn from intact indigenous cultures that still honor the feminine. One example is the Andean culture of the Quechua people. In their language, the earth is referred to as Pachamama, which literally translates as "Mother World." Spiritual teacher Javier Regueiro, who lives in Peru and has apprenticed with various teachers in the Iquitos and Pucallpa areas, explained to me, "To the Quechua, the planet is perceived and experienced as a quintessentially feminine living organism. She is a passionately joyful, generous mother, who nurtures and nourishes us. Through her ceaseless process of reproduction, she showers us with air, water, food, and beauty. She is portrayed as an image of plenty. She is abundance itself, forever in creation, transforming and evolving."

Once you embrace Mother Earth as sacred, you can trust that your body is sacred too. The prevailing religious indoctrination of "transcendence" teaches us that we experience the divine by transcending the physical world, which again alienates us from our bodies and most often leads us to believe that they are dirty and sinful and that their desires are depraved. However, a return to the spiritual values of earth-based cultures reminds us of "immanence," the understanding that we experience the divine through the physical world. Immanence exalts the feminine and teaches us to have an appreciation for the natural creatures that are our bodies.

You can think of your struggle with food, weight, and body image as a call to return to the belief in immanence and its feminine values. As Javier Regueiro teaches, unlike masculine consciousness—which is about the survival of the fittest and praising those who make it to the top—feminine consciousness, or mother consciousness, is about the inclusion of all beings. When you start living from this consciousness, you will no longer be able to neglect your body's needs for fresh, healthy food, physical activity, loving relationships, and creative and sexual expression. Never again will you be capable of being a cold, unfeeling master of your body, inflicting junk food upon her simply because it is an easy fix for hunger.

PLEASURE BITE

To remind you of the intimate connection between your female animal and Mother Earth, take a silent walk in nature. Walk in a forest, stroll along a river, or meander through a park. Open your senses to the wonders of the physical world around you, as well as the magic of your own physical body.

REUNITING WITH YOUR WILD DESIRES

What's most threatening to some women about my philosophy of acknowledging our bodies as animals are the untamed, undomesticated desires of animals. Where it was once part of the Great Mystery that certain things remain unknowable, in a mind-centered culture, everything unknown is a threat. Our culture fears our wild side, associating wildness with savage, unrestrained behavior.

If you accept that your body is a wise, decision-making female animal that instinctively knows what to eat to lose weight, then you must trust your wild, raw instincts in all areas of life. You can't selectively trust your desires with food yet doubt them when it comes to sex or relationships. That's why Pleasurable Weight Loss is much more than a diet or even a lifestyle shift. This approach is about the radical act of trusting not only your pleasure but also your wildness in every dimension of life.

The final hurdle that marked my liberation from ten years of struggle with emotional eating was a willingness to embrace all of my desires, no matter how simple or wild. I was brought up to think that desire was dangerous. To avoid being reprimanded by my parents, as much as possible I hid my desires—my secret trysts with food and my explorations of my sexuality. But when

I realized that my body is an animal with innate desires that are good and wise, I was finally able to put this conflict behind me. When I gave myself permission to trust my desires, to my absolute surprise, my body's response to the question, "What do you desire to eat?" wasn't "forbidden foods" like ice cream or cake. Instead, she said in a loud voice, "I'd like some salmon, brown rice, and vegetables." This is when I realized that I could trust my body's desires and that they would guide me to heal my weight issues and my relationship with food.

PLEASURE PRACTICE
What Do You Desire?

Write a list of your deepest desires. What do you really want in life? What do you hunger for? What does your heart most desire? Your body most desire? Your soul most desire?

These desires don't need to be practical, easily fulfilled, or socially acceptable. They simply need to be the desires that live deep within you and call to you. These can be sexual desires, financial desires, lifestyle desires, emotional desires, desires for food, people, places, and forbidden desires—anything you can imagine. As you write this list, free yourself to be real and honest, raw and open.

Accept your desires as your own. Read your list every day. Breathe your desires in. The secret to reaping the most benefit from your desires is to relish not only their fulfillment but also the experience of yearning itself. Even if you don't know how you will accomplish your desires, let them live inside you as sources of pleasure in and of themselves.

PLEASURE BITE

Every day is an occasion for a dance break. All it takes is dancing full out to one song to get you connected to your animal. Pick a song (or three!), and as you dance, appreciate your body. You have been blessed by the gift of a human life. Scientists say that the statistical probability of being born a human (as opposed to a turtle or a tree) is one in 400 trillion. Dance with gratitude to remind yourself how deeply fortunate you are.

PLEASURABLE EATING PRACTICE 1
Checking In with Your Animal

The first Pleasurable Eating Practice connects you with your body before you eat. Imagine you are going to share a meal with a friend and that friend is your female animal. As you sit down to eat, ask your animal how she's feeling. Be present to her desires. Does she have any needs, such as a glass of water or a more comfortable sitting posture?

Then, ask her what she would like to eat. Listen carefully to what she has to say, and base your food choices on a collaboration between your body and mind. Your animal may request some of the foods that your mind fears, such as potato chips or cupcakes. When this happens, don't stress: feeling ashamed about her cravings is more harmful than eating the food itself. If after listening closely to her desire, you truly want it, go ahead. Locate what you want to eat. Choose the highest-quality version of that food, made with the best and freshest ingredients.

Now that you have reconnected with your animal and begun to respect and pay attention to your instinctive feminine desires, the next step on our journey of pleasurable weight loss is to become fluent in your body's native language, which is pleasure.

Let your desire for pleasure—your desire for feeling good—
be your only guiding light.

ABRAHAM HICKS

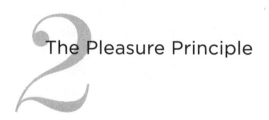

The Pleasure Principle

WHEN I WAS STRUGGLING with my weight and my relationship with food, I was convinced that having too much
pleasure was the cause of my problem. Throughout my life, I've
always desired to live every day to the fullest, and I've embraced
all of life's pleasures with gusto, including food. When I was a
binge-eater, I would indulge in my favorite foods, like cheese,
bread, cookies, cakes, ice cream, and chocolate. I was ashamed of
my relationship with food, and I hated the effect it was having
on my protruding waistline. So why did I keep coming back for
more? The answer was simple. Because eating these foods gave
me pleasure.

So it was easy for me to surmise that pleasure was the root of
my problem. I thought that if I just weren't so compelled by this
darn craving for pleasure, I wouldn't be overeating, and I wouldn't
be overweight. Instead, I'd be thin and beautiful! I was suspicious and distrustful of pleasure. I blamed my desires for being the
nefarious force that caused me to eat the foods that in my head I
knew I shouldn't. Regardless of my mind's opinion and no matter

how much I tried to control the situation, my body was oblivious and seemed unstoppably attracted to pleasure's call.

I often lamented whether it was a sick joke nature played on humanity: for pleasure to feel so good but leave unpleasant consequences behind. Why is cheese so delicious if we are to be punished with weight gain when we eat it? What I didn't realize at the time was that I had it all backwards. My problem was not that I was having too much pleasure; my problem was that I wasn't having enough! I'd been raised to think of pleasure as an occasional reward for hard work, and my life reflected that belief. Whether it was school, sports, music, or one of my multiple jobs, I was a poster child for working hard. Aside from my shame-filled encounters with food and sex, pleasure was an afterthought at best. For me, pleasure was something that had to be earned.

The truth is that pleasure is a biological requirement. Contrary to what society would have us believe, pleasure, like breathing, is not a luxury but a non-negotiable need. "Pleasure in its essence is a guide to health. The reason things feel good is that there is an evolutionary reason to seek them out," says Christopher Ryan.

All living creatures have obeyed one shared evolutionary principle since they first appeared on the planet: seek pleasure and avoid pain. From the simple amoeba to the complex human being, this mechanism has been the evolutionary compass safely guiding every life form on our planet to evolve to where it is today.

For example, when our ancestors discovered fire and its accompanying benefits of cooking food, providing warmth, and deterring predators, they knew they had stumbled upon a good thing. You can bet they weren't sitting around moralizing, "Well, do you think we should really be enjoying this? Is this too much pleasure for our own good? Will this take the edge off our work ethic?" Hell no. Their instinctive wisdom told them that the pleasure of sustenance, warmth, and protection would support their survival. At the same time, the instinct to avoid pain would have taught them, "The flames are hot. Don't sit too close, for we will be burned." In other words, our ancestors were successful because they paid attention to pleasure and avoided pain. You are here because your ancestors were diligent pleasure seekers. As self-love expert Michel Madie says, "It was pleasurable to procreate, pleasurable to eat, pleasurable to feed children from our breasts, and to teach them about the world. It was pleasurable to belong within a society and to protect each other."

Today, pleasure continues to be a necessary component for our survival, particularly when it comes to food. Science has found that when we eat with pleasure, we help our metabolism, which makes digestion more efficient and assists with weight loss. The simple act of eating releases feel-good biochemicals known as endorphins. That fact alone indicates that from an evolutionary view, eating is meant to be inherently pleasurable. Endorphins also stimulate metabolism, and as Marc David explains in his book *The Slow Down Diet,* the same biochemical that makes us feel good when we eat burns body fat, too. So when we put this all together, the lesson is: when eating becomes more pleasurable, we heighten our capacity to lose weight. Isn't that fantastic?

Tragically, we've been so deeply indoctrinated to mistrust our pleasure with food that when we do enjoy eating the foods we love most, many of us feel ashamed about it. We fear that our cravings signify an inner weakness that should be controlled. But food is meant to be relished and eaten with gusto, not with reserve or analysis, as science shows. Feeling guilty while we eat promotes weight gain, but allowing ourselves to be ignited by the pleasure of food literally flips on the switch that fully engages our metabolism.

Once I came to understand the importance of pleasure, I could appreciate the hidden wisdom behind my eating binges. I had been operating as if pleasure were bad and hard work were good, and I focused all my available energy on productive achievements. I did not know that by neglecting to attend to my pleasure, I was denying a force stronger than my mind could withstand.

GREET YOUR DAY WITH PLEASURE

You can use the willpower of your mind to discipline your animal and push the temptation of pleasure away for a time. But here's the part that traditional diets overlook: at some point, when your mind is exhausted and can no longer maintain its role as the security guard against pleasure, it inevitably falls asleep on the job, and your animal, aware that the coast is clear, will steal into action. Exhausting your willpower can occur as early as breakfast, and when it does, compulsive eating begins. In the moment, it looks like pleasure is the "problem." But dig a little deeper, and you'll see that it's the rejection of pleasure that has set the stage for compulsive eating. If your animal doesn't get pleasure in a healthy way, she will take it—with or without your approval—in whatever way she can. You do have a choice: healthy pleasure or unhealthy pleasure. The only outcome that's not an option is no pleasure.

Imagine greeting your day with an appreciation of pleasure as a biological requirement, a wise guiding force in your life. Before jumping on your email, reading the newspaper, or racing to fulfill someone else's needs, you give yourself a few minutes of pleasure. You put on the stereo and dance, or you meditate and invite your mind to rest and relax. Maybe you gaze out your window at the clouds or listen to the birds. Even if you have only a few minutes, you use them wisely to fill your pleasure tank.

Imagine seizing every opportunity to pepper your day with pleasure. You wear an outfit you love. During your commute you listen to an audiobook that expands your mind. You make a point to eat lunch in a tranquil environment. When you hit your mid-afternoon slump, instead of buckling down with a cup of coffee in hand, like a weapon ready for battle, you take a walk to refresh yourself. After all, productivity experts agree that sacrificing pleasure in the name of time management and efficiency has the opposite effect: it actually slows us down. On the way home, you pick up a bunch of flowers for your kitchen, simply because they give you delight, and when you're home, you phone your girlfriend for some nourishing girl talk.

Now, how would you feel at the end of such a day? My guess is that you'd feel energized and rewarded, and you'd feel like you matter. In small ways throughout the day, you tended to your body's biological requirement for pleasure. Would you still feel the call of the cookie jar? Maybe. But with the understanding that your body is an animal evolution designed to be a pleasure-seeking creature, the allure of the cookie will be seen through a new perspective. Instead of feeling guilty for wanting a sweet treat, you will feel innocent. This conscious shift—removing the guilt and shame about pleasure and instead embracing it—is where the magic of Pleasurable Weight Loss kicks into gear.

Liberated from shame's grip, you are free to unpack the layers of your cookie craving.

Instead of rejecting your desire with an iron fist or being blindly dragged into the pantry against your better judgment, you are able to approach the situation with curiosity. When you lead with curiosity as opposed to anger, guilt, or shame, you'll find that you have at your disposal the luxury of choice. If a cookie is what your body really wants, then you have the freedom to locate the best possible cookie you can get your hands on—perhaps an organic, whole-grain cookie, made with maple syrup, instead of a white-sugar cookie. And when you eat the cookie, you do so with curiosity, and you savor every bite as if it were the first cookie you'd ever eaten. Maybe you discover you don't actually enjoy the cookie, so you put it down and seek pleasure elsewhere.

Perhaps your pleasure craving would be equally satisfied by a good belly laugh, which you enjoy while watching a funny YouTube video or chatting with a loved one. If you are at home when you hear the cookie jar calling, your options may be more plentiful. Maybe a hot bath, a foot rub, or even a catnap on the couch would please your animal. I've never met a woman who resorted to overeating when presented with a buffet of pleasure options. It's when we deny our natural need for pleasure that we close the doors of our perception and overlook healthier options for pleasure that promote weight loss.

Pleasure is so powerful it can revitalize your metabolism. You'll find that when you're going through a relaxed period in your life and you're in the flow, you'll lose weight without even trying. This tells us not to focus on losing weight directly but to address it indirectly instead. Sustainable weight loss comes not through restricting what you do or eat but by expanding the areas in your life that give you pleasure.

When you deprive yourself of pleasure with food, chances are you are also depriving yourself of pleasure in other areas of your life. It's likely that you are also missing out on needed touch, movement, and sensual and sexual satisfaction. As pleasure expert Tonya Leigh says, "You need to diversify your pleasure portfolio." If too much of your body's pleasure quota is invested in food, then you're not investing in pleasure wisely. The pleasure you seek from food then becomes exaggerated because your animal is trying to tell you that she is in extreme need. So you seek intensely sweet, salty, or greasy foods, or you drink lots of alcohol in an attempt to fill your pleasure quota all at once. But when you have access to a variety of pleasure sources, your animal will be satisfied with the subtler tastes of natural foods, and refined junk foods will actually lose their appeal.

PLEASURE PRACTICE
What Brings You Pleasure?

For me, a treat always used to be something to eat. But now I know that there are infinite sources of delight other than food, such as beauty, comfort, adventure, companionship, mischief, sensuality, fun, and play. Once you are willing to research what brings you pleasure, you'll find you have at your disposal a wide array of pleasure sources beyond the predictable and easy quick fix of food. True pleasure can be found everywhere. You just need to allow space for it.

Write a list of everything that has brought you pleasure in your life. Include people, places, foods, erotic experiences, feelings, thoughts, things, and situations. Describe how you found them, what they have meant to you, how they have helped or healed you. Let the list grow by adding to it every time you discover something new that brings you pleasure.

Also, brainstorm a list of every pleasure imaginable—not only pleasures you have known but also those you dream of. Which forms of pleasure can you incorporate right now?

ENJOYING PLEASURE IS AN ART
The pleasurable approach to weight loss requires you to consider pleasure an art. It's time to become a connoisseur of true pleasure. If you blindly follow the pleasures TV ads suggest, you risk ending up with a sick, unhappy, and overweight animal. That's because modern pleasures can be confusing to our bodies; our pleasure instincts were instilled in more innocent, ancient times. Your body's intense response to the pleasure of sweet tastes evolved in a world where sweet foods were rare. Honey, for example, could

only be had at the risk of encountering a swarm of angry bees. Indulging in honey was not an option. Our instincts were also wired in an environment where all food was natural and organic.

Today, the same reward system that motivated us to search out the sweets of the natural world is operating in a new environment. We are like moths that once flew in night skies lit only by stars. Their once elegant nocturnal survival strategy has been undermined by the invention of electricity. Every porch light is a survival hazard for a moth. Today, we find ourselves in an era of grocery stores that can easily satisfy our cravings with a jar of honey or a bag of candy. Our primal reward system is still being activated, but the ease of access to foods and food products has transformed our attraction to sweets from a reward to a liability. Still worse, corporations spend billions of dollars on advertising to entice us to crave processed foods, corrupting our natural instincts for pleasure. The only way to protect your animal is to become consciously aware.

So where does this conundrum leave you? Suspicious of pleasure again? No. That reaction is the mistake millions of women make when they continue to reject pleasure because they fear the consequences and complexities. On the contrary, this situation illuminates the need to become a connoisseur of true pleasure, someone who can distinguish between high-quality and low-quality pleasures, someone who knows her female animal deserves only the best.

A connoisseur of true pleasure knows that pleasure is more than a momentary burst on the taste buds. She embraces pleasure with a democratic attitude, which means she recognizes that all parts of her deserve pleasure. Besides, the truth is that when we overeat or eat foods laden with chemicals, we may stimulate the tongue, but we don't make our animals feel good in other ways. Overeating can cause a bellyache or a headache or make us feel spaced out or fatigued. If you're honest with yourself, you've already realized that overeating doesn't actually make you feel good for long. As author Geneen Roth says, "It is when pleasure ends that overeating begins."

If you pay close attention to your pleasure as you eat, as a connoisseur would, then you'll notice when the experience ceases to be pleasurable and instead becomes dull and automatic. This shift indicates that you have crossed the line and moved from eating in accord with your animal's needs and desires to unconscious overeating. No matter to what degree you may have convinced yourself that overeating gives you pleasure, when experienced from your animal's perspective, you know that's not true. All animals in nature eat just the right amount—and not more.

Once you can discern the beginning and the end of a pleasurable experience by staying present, you will become a true pleasure connoisseur. And then, you will be able to respond to your desires without worrying that they will lead you down an ultimately painful path.

Give yourself the most luxurious bath you can create. Light candles and put on your favorite relaxing music. Fill the tub high and add scented oil—perhaps lavender or ylang-ylang. Feel decadent by adding fresh flower petals to the water. Let yourself feel indulged.

TRUE PLEASURE VS. COUNTERFEIT PLEASURE

A pleasure connoisseur can differentiate two types of pleasure that others confuse: true pleasure and counterfeit pleasure. True pleasure is like life itself—it is sustainable. It can be enjoyed without compromising your ability to have more in the future. For example, think about the way you feel after eating a juicy, fresh peach versus the way you feel after binging on chocolate cake. True pleasure is not what sends us scurrying compulsively back for more. What's more, the mind-set of true pleasure is rooted in a belief in both an abundant universe and our ability to manifest our desires—so we're able to enjoy an experience without the stress of worrying whether more will be available down the line. True pleasure gives us this lesson: when you're no longer shamelessly enjoying the experience, it is no longer a pleasure.

Love coach Annie Lalla teaches that true pleasure answers "yes" to this filter question: Will this experience give me pleasure now, in an hour, in a day, in a week, in a month, and in a year? If not, you are looking at a counterfeit pleasure. Annie Lalla says, "Counterfeit pleasure occurs when the natural, useful, life-preserving pleasure reward system is co-opted by a shorter-term compulsive strategy that gives a short-term hit instead of a long-term gain. It no longer serves your development or survival; it actually compromises it."

For example, the counterfeit pleasure of gorging on even your favorite food may leave you feeling terrible as soon as an hour later (and we all know where it leads over time). True pleasure is the ice cream cone you savored on a hot day, which leaves a fond memory you can enjoy for years. Counterfeit pleasure is polishing off an entire pint of ice cream in one sitting, which leaves a sugar hangover and a stew of private shame.

Counterfeit pleasure is tied to compulsive behavior. In an effort to again feel the reward you initially felt from food, alcohol, shopping, or sex, you return to that same experience, but each time you return, you need a little more of whatever was pleasurable to get the same feeling of satisfaction. What's more, even when you repeat the event, it doesn't make you feel good. Someone with a food compulsion doesn't actually enjoy eating the very same cake she can't stop herself from finishing.

If your desire for whatever it is you want to eat has a loose, unattached energy, you are not under the grip of a food compulsion. True pleasure is not compulsive; counterfeit pleasure is. Whenever I refer to pleasure in this book, I am referring only to true pleasure. As you develop your wisdom and better understand pleasure's impact across time in your own life, you will be better equipped to distinguish between true pleasure and counterfeit pleasure. When you learn to tell the difference and fill your days with all kinds of true pleasures, you will see that your life flourishes and your body lightens up as a natural side effect.

PLEASURE AND ADDICTION

Pleasure and addiction are distinct but can be confused for the same thing. Here's the difference: pleasure is the comfortable feeling of choosing from a series of options, while addiction is a compulsive feeling that narrows your choices. Addiction stems from a negative judgment on pleasure. When we don't accept our natural desire for pleasure but instead judge it and relegate it to the shadows, we plant a seed for addiction. Your animal's healthy pleasure-seeking instinct is forced into secret, guilt-ridden, dysfunctional behaviors that are ultimately damaging, unlike the healing nature of true pleasure. When we are ashamed of pleasure, we go through motions that are meant to give us pleasure but without truly experiencing it. Because we don't get what we need out of the experience, we seek more of it, and so the cycle of addiction goes on.

Addictions are counterfeit pleasures. Pleasure may be the impulse that had you take the first bite or the first sip, but by the time you've eaten your way into a food coma or drunk yourself into oblivion, consumption is no longer pleasurable. What's driving you to keep eating or drinking is shame. That's when you're thinking even while you're eating: "I shouldn't be doing this. I know where this goes. I'll never lose weight. I'll always be fat and disgusting."

Shame and pleasure cannot co-exist, nor can guilt and pleasure. The whole idea of "a guilty pleasure" is shame-making dressed up in disguise. If you are feeling guilty about an experience—even if you appear to be having a ball on the outside—at the deepest level you will be compromising how much of a good time you can really have. When shame commands your attention, at least a part of your awareness leaves the food or drink in your mouth to attend to the thoughts in your head. As a result, your female animal is not able to fully experience the pleasure she was hoping for when she sent the signal to eat or drink. In this kind of situation, listen to the voice of your female animal instead of focusing on your shame. Always check in with your female animal to determine what is truly pleasurable for her—bite by bite by bite—and you will be able to eat free of shame because at your core you will know you have listened to her true needs.

PLEASURE BITE

Choose the fruit you find most sensuous (for me, it's a juicy mango) and treat yourself to a sensual eating ritual. Prepare the fruit, place it on a beautiful plate, and then blindfold yourself. Let your animal loose as you engage your senses while eating. Savor the smell, texture, and taste of this ripe gift from nature.

GETTING THE MOST PLEASURE FROM FOOD

It's time to throw away the punishing diet mentality and to embrace the discipline of pleasure. Commit to fully enjoying every pleasurable bite of your food, whether it's your favorite chocolate, a sun-ripened strawberry, or wholesome beans and rice. This is the time to experience freedom and self-love with food. Eat foods that delight you, and make every meal a ritual for honoring the divine within you.

The pleasurable strategies we're exploring will help you relax, and when you're relaxed, it will be easier to have the awareness to make healthy choices that will prevent unwanted weight gain. What's more, you'll find that eating healthy foods is a true pleasure: you'll enjoy eating them, and you'll feel great afterwards.

And remember that the more you enjoy what brings you pleasure in all areas of your life, the easier it will be to eat better. When I was a compulsive eater, every five minutes my head was back in the fridge because I was bored: I was working too hard and didn't make it a point to access true pleasure. Even if your life appears to be okay and you are sitting comfortably at home doing nothing, if you are not fulfilled in life, you will turn to food to fill the gap. When you are fulfilled, you don't need the compensation overeating provides. Let your desire to lose weight and have a peaceful relationship with food be the fuel that motivates you to have the discipline to bring pleasure to everything.

PLEASURABLE EATING PRACTICE 2
Enhance Your Eating Environment

Making each meal a pleasurable experience contributes to your digestive power and calorie-burning efficiency. Pay attention to your eating environment. Create a space that is conducive to your enjoyment. If you are eating at home, make it a point to sit at a table. Turn off the television and computer and put away other devices and distractions. Clear any clutter. Serve your food on dishes that you find attractive. You might even light a candle to symbolize your presence to the food at hand. Create as relaxing and pleasurable an eating space as possible.

TRUE PLEASURE REQUIRES PRESENCE

When it comes to experiencing true pleasure, the present moment is the place to be. Thinking about the pleasures you've had in the past or pleasures you intend to have in the future taps you only into the concept of pleasure. True pleasure exists in the present. Unless you are present, you are not fully experiencing pleasure.

Being present is a skill many spiritual traditions encourage. Now before you yawn, "Oh, here comes the mindfulness lecture," let me assure you that being present is not just about piously watching your breath while sitting on a meditation cushion. Being fully present means being present to your thoughts, emotions, and body at the same time, and it is the secret to unlocking a pleasure-filled existence, including a slim figure and a peaceful relationship with food.

From an evolutionary view, once upon a time there was no choice but to live in the present—that's all our brains could handle. But as we developed centers in our brains that grant the perception of passing time, we were given the ability to place our attention on the past or to think about the future. And while there's nothing wrong with reminiscing or with dreaming about the future, being engaged in the present moment is the whole point of life.

Take the example of my client Lisa, a successful entrepreneur who lived a dream life. She had a great guy, a newborn baby, and her own business. But she told me in despair, "I'm a sugar addict." Once I taught her the practice of being truly present while eating, however, Lisa reported back to me, "I've realized I don't even like sugar that much. I feel awful after I eat it, and when I'm really present with the taste, I notice it's not as delicious as I thought."

Think of true pleasure as meditation in disguise. Whereas the practice of meditation focuses the mind on your breath, a mantra, or a creative visualization, the practice of pleasure requires you to be aware of what you are experiencing through the senses. No matter how much your mind tries to convince you you're having a ball, unless your consciousness is present with your pleasure at the sensory level—seeing, tasting, smelling, touching, and hearing—you're not fully deriving pleasure from the experience.

And this is where things get interesting. Because your body has been programmed over time to seek pleasure, if you are not present when you eat, you will miss out on the benefits of the pleasure that nature intended—which includes the signal to the brain that you are full and satisfied. This is why, no matter how much you eat, unless you pay attention, it will always feel like something is missing, and you won't feel satiated.

Imagine you have something on your mind and you crave the support of a caring friend. So there you are, pouring your heart out to her, but your friend is not paying attention. She is checking her text messages, posting a quick Facebook update, or absent-mindedly staring out the window. No matter how passionately or clearly you express yourself, if your friend isn't present with you, you'll feel your needs weren't met, and you'll seek out someone else to talk to, someone who will be present.

In the same way, if you gobble down your food while mul-titasking—whether you're watching TV, surfing the Web, talking on the phone, or distracted by something happening outside of you—you lose awareness of what's taking place in your mouth and belly, which causes your body to respond by signaling that you need more. It's as if your body is saying, "I didn't see anything, smell anything, taste anything, or feel anything. It seems like noth-ing happened. I must need to eat more." When I was overeating, I was always baffled by the quantities of food I could eat and still be hungry. Now I understand why: I wasn't present when I was eating. When we're present, pleasure does not have to turn into overindulgence. You can feel great during and after the experience.

Every single moment in life is an opportunity to practice the skill of being present. Noticing the texture of clothes against your skin, the scent of the outdoors, the taste of your lover's kiss, the sound of laughter, and the sight of a setting sun—all give you an occasion to hone your senses to the present moment. Pay atten-tion to the tiny moments of pleasure each day provides that can so easily be overlooked.

If you go through your life numb to the delights of the sun's caress on your skin, the deep warmth of a hug, or the toe-tingling exhilaration of great sex, it's going to take a lot more effort to become aware of edible pleasures. But if you proactively heighten your awareness of the pleasures life bestows on you on a daily basis, then being attuned to pleasure while you eat will become second nature. The more you hone your ability to notice all pleasure, the more aware you will be of the true pleasure you receive from eating—and the less likely you will be to overeat or to reach for unhealthy foods that hold the promise of pleasure but do not deliver.

How do we learn to be present? It sounds simple, but being present is a learned art. And it's never too late to start learning. Here are a few techniques to begin:

- A universal tool for becoming present is paying attention to your breath. Notice it flow in and out. Meditation is a great practice for noticing the breath, as is yoga, tai chi, swimming, and other awareness-based physical practices that synchronize movement with the breath.

- Blink your eyes. The intentional act of blinking your eyes brings you to the present moment because you are bringing your consciousness to your body. This is a useful tool when you find yourself zoning out of a conversation and want to discreetly bring your focus back to the present.

- Scan through each of your senses. One by one, bring your attention to the five senses. As you focus on each sense, let the others fall away. For example, if you smell a flower, close your eyes, breathe in its fragrance, and then let your mind rest.

- Look out at what's before you. So often our eyes are open and we are technically seeing, but without our presence, we are not really taking in what is before us. With this practice, you look out at the world to consciously take in what you see before you.

- Take in your outer experience and your inner experience at once. Shine your awareness on your external environment while you continue to maintain a connection to what you feel within yourself.

TO BE PRESENT IS TO BE GROUNDED

Another way to describe being present is being grounded. I first learned the phrase *to be grounded* from an earthy woman who enjoyed walking barefoot. As I got to know her, she revealed that one of her daily practices was paying attention to being grounded, and I immediately loved the sound of it.

When you are grounded, you are completely aware of what's happening, both in yourself and in your environment. You are present to your body's sensations. Your face softens, your breath relaxes, and you sit more comfortably. Your voice becomes clearer. You feel like a queen—powerful, confident, wise, and authentic. When you are grounded, you can discern the difference between hunger and habit, between the true need of your animal and an old pattern that no longer serves you. I used to feel anxious and uncertain about what to eat, and I reacted by overeating everything. I wasn't grounded, and so I was unable to distinguish my true needs.

My client Patricia was troubled by her compulsive eating and weight. I could immediately sense that she was not grounded and was trying to ground herself by eating. She told me that she didn't identify with her body; she viewed herself as a head on a stick. To help her create a new connection to her body we explored pleasurable options for becoming grounded that didn't involve food—applying lotion, daily stretching, weekly massage, walks in the park, and visits to local hot springs. As she spent more time being present with the physical sensations she experienced during these activities, she began to connect with her body, her animal. Before, Patricia would eat her way through a box of cookies in an unconscious blur, but now that she was grounded, she could divert her attention away from the pantry. Without feeling that she was restricting herself, she started to lose weight.

You know you aren't grounded when you are scattered, easily distracted, forgetful, clumsy, unsure of yourself, or anxious. Physically you may feel jittery, wired, or have a nervous pit in your stomach. These are your animal's signals that she needs to ground. Unless you respond to these signals with healthy ways to ground, you are vulnerable to unconsciously turning to food, as the density of food in your body can be a grounding force.

When you are grounded, the whirlwind of thoughts in your head slows down, and everything becomes quiet and clear. Neither thoughts about the past nor worries about the future affect you. Fear and anxiety dissipate, and a sensation of being connected with an endless source of energy is present. Grounding allows you to experience the stillness in which you can hear your body's signals loud and clear—so much so, that your body's wisdom can no longer be ignored.

So how do you become present and grounded in the moment when you are reaching for the cookie jar? Dance instructor Tenley Wallace shared this exercise with me. Let's imagine you have a mid-afternoon snack habit, and you're stuck in a pattern of eating more cookies than you know is ideal and pleasurable for your body. The first step is to notice exactly what you are doing in that moment. Watch your hand reaching out to merge with that cookie. Now, purposefully bring your attention to your hand and bring it back to the body. Start to consciously lengthen your inhalations and exhalations, and start to perceive the sensations in your environment in that moment. Notice how the rest of your system responds to your deeper breathing. Soften your knees, relax your pelvis, and feel your feet. Then with awareness, send the breath up your body and then down your body. Staying with the breath, take inventory of what is going on for you.

Once you are grounded, you can get clear on what your true need is. Maybe you really do want a cookie (but not the entire box), or maybe what you need is a drink of water, a deep breath, a walk, a dance break, or some chamomile tea.

PLEASURE PRACTICE
Get Grounded

One of the most pleasurable places to get grounded is outdoors. If you can, do this exercise barefoot, feeling the grass, soil, sand, or rocks beneath your feet. Feel the wind or the gentle breeze against your skin. Stand with your weight evenly distributed and close your eyes. Imagine that you are an ancient tree, firmly rooted and connected with Mother Earth. Pay attention to the bottoms of your feet and how they connect to the earth. Bend your knees slightly to increase the sensation of the earth pressing up as you press down toward her. Begin to take deep breaths into your lower belly and visualize roots growing out of the soles of your feet, down through the earth, penetrating deep into the earth's core. See the roots become stronger and thicker as they grow ever more deeply into the earth, all the way to her molten core. Once you feel connected with the earth through these roots, open your eyes. Start to walk slowly and visualize your roots emerging from each foot as it returns to the ground.

YOU ARE THE AUTHOR OF YOUR LIFE

When you are grounded, you can make the empowered choices that will support the weight loss you want. The secret again is to respect the instincts and desires of your animal. Without listening to your animal, you will be victim to your addictions, expectations, and outside definitions of what is good and bad to eat, as well as what is or is not pleasurable.

Most women are raised, subtly or not so subtly, to assume a victim mentality. We've become accustomed to the internal refrain, especially in the realm of weight loss: "Poor me. Why is this happening to me?" In every "poor me" story, there's a victim and a perpetrator. The victim is the "goodie," and the perpetrator is the "baddie." When it comes to the struggle with weight loss, emotional eating, and bad body image, it can feel like your body is the perpetrator, the enemy within: "Why is it doing this to me?"

It's easy to jump to the conclusion that you have been wronged. And while you cannot be in control of every circumstance or outcome, there's nothing more deadening to pleasure than dwelling on all the ways life treats you unfairly. Not only does this mindset make you uninviting to be around, but it also has a detrimental effect on your weight.

When you hold a victim mentality, needless to say, it is a stressful experience. We will look more closely at the biochemistry of stress in the next chapter. For now, know that when we experience stress, the body represses metabolism, which encourages weight gain. Who knew that feeling sorry for yourself could be a weight loss hazard? Gaining weight can make you feel all the more victimized by circumstances. Until you escape what I call the "Infinite Lack of Accountability Loop," you can be forever caught in a vicious weight gain cycle.

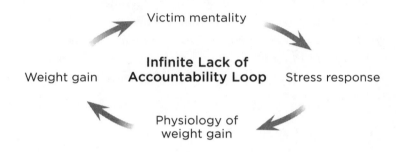

figure 1

But when you have the right tools, you will have the power to control how you respond to life's challenges. To escape this loop requires learning to step back from a situation to see things differently. When you embrace the role of a victim, you will always find supporting evidence that the world really has wronged you in one way or another. "Yes, your boss is a jerk," a friend will console you, thinking she is supporting you, but in effect unwittingly enabling your victim game. The magic happens when you have the courage to look at the situation through a different lens.

While you may feel certain that in a given situation, you are clearly the victim and the other is the perpetrator, this perspective depends on whose shoulder you are looking over. For example, if a friend cancels a lunch date, you might respond as the victim, thinking your friend is the perpetrator: "You don't care about me. You're not prioritizing our friendship." But when you make her guilty, she experiences you as the perpetrator and herself as the victim. By allowing yourself to feel like a victim, you necessarily brand someone else a perpetrator. This dance can go on and on for a lifetime. "I'm the victim in this situation," says one; "No, no, I'm the victim," retorts the other. Although at first glance the roles of victim and perpetrator appear to be worlds apart, a closer look shows they are two sides of the same coin: both victim and perpetrator refuse to take responsibility. In fact, serial victims might be the worst perpetrators because they deny their part in creating situations.

The way out of the cycle is to adopt a new perspective: accountability. Being accountable is not to be confused with accounting—it has nothing to do with numbers. It's all about storytelling. Being accountable means acknowledging your dual role as both the author and the protagonist of your life story. Usually we identify only as the protagonist, but the magic that fuels pleasurable weight loss happens when you realize you are also the author holding the pen. You are writing the script that you, the main character, are living out.

Now you may be thinking, why the heck would I write a script where I am overweight, compulsive with food, and grossed out by my own body? It's a great question. But whatever the reason, in this moment, you get to choose your answers to the questions: Who am I as a human being, and who do I want to become? This is what it means to be accountable.

If you dislike your body right now or any aspect of your life, it means there's always a little more accountability you can take. The secret is to take just enough to get what you want. Taken to an extreme, being accountable can make you feel that everything is your fault. That is not my intention. You are not solely responsible for global warming, for example, but you are responsible for your own satisfaction with your life and your body.

Leadership advisor Bryan Franklin describes the act of moving from victim/perpetrator to accountability as, "eating a shit sandwich" (nice visual, eh?). Eating a shit sandwich is clearly not a pleasant experience. It means admitting you played a role in creating the situation you find yourself in and owning your ability to create something different. Although eating a shit sandwich may not be tasty, stewing in the juices of victimhood is far more toxic. Whenever you catch yourself looping on the "poor me" thought, remind yourself, "I'm not a victim; I'm creating this."

Bryan then suggests asking yourself, "What would be the most entertaining next move in the direction of my desired outcome?" This question is meant to inspire you to author an interesting story for yourself. Stories have a very powerful effect on the mind. The story you internalize about yourself becomes the story of who you are. This is the immense responsibility and gift of becoming accountable: you realize you have the power to shape your destiny.

When you find yourself in the victim role, convinced that you have been wronged, it's useful to ask yourself, "What am I getting out of this situation?" Usually the payoff for the victim is the satisfaction of holding the high moral ground. It feels so good to be the one who is "right" that we are willing to play the part of the one who has been "wronged." However, when you release your perpetrators from their roles by becoming accountable, you may relinquish the high moral ground of the victim, but you return to an equal footing. Whatever you feel you may be losing, the wins are greater. By becoming accountable, you acknowledge that you are a free and sovereign being, creating her own reality. And there is no better feeling than that!

Feeling like a victim occurs when your boundaries have been disregarded or you never established them in the first place. In either case, instead of seeking an apology from the perpetrator, you can shift from a victim mind-set to a mind-set of accountability with Bryan's mantra: "Thank you for showing me where I didn't have boundaries." When you reframe what you previously felt was a violation against you as a lesson in boundaries, you become a player in the experience and take some responsibility for what unfolds.

When my client Dara first came to me, she told me how she sacrificed her needs for others. In the story of her life, she was always the martyr or the victim. Her days were filled with compromises she resented making. But when she realized how her victim mind-set was holding her back in all areas of her life, including weight loss, she knew she had to change. I taught her that to reframe every situation in which she felt like a victim was an opportunity to be more honest with herself and with others. By setting better boundaries, Dara didn't have to quiet her resentment with food. When she stopped being a victim, Dara's clothes became looser, and her life became more fulfilling, too.

Even in the worst situations, owning your sovereignty triggers the relaxation response. By changing your perception from victim to creator of your life, you let go of the bonds that were holding you back and thereby redirect your life experience. It's no surprise that this condition needs to be met to achieve weight loss.

Whenever there is a victim dynamic, it's natural to start looking for a hero, someone who will come to our rescue. With weight loss, you might have hoped that the latest diet or workout would be that hero. But the real hero lies within. Once you become accountable, you'll realize that no one, no diet, no nothing can save you from your struggles with food and weight. You are the creator of your reality. It's up to you to become your heroine.

In science, such accountability and authorship are referred to as self-regulation, where you learn to influence the nervous system in order to create an alert yet calm and relaxed body-mind state. When you take radical responsibility for your emotional state, you learn to create effective strategies to soothe your nervous system so that you don't have to turn to food to change your state. This requires listening to your animal, being grounded, and creating healthy boundaries.

PLEASURE PRACTICE
Accountability in Action

Scan your life for the areas where you feel most frustrated, disappointed, stuck, or victimized. On a piece of paper, divide the page into two columns. In the column on the left, write down all the places where you identify yourself as a victim. Then reflect on how feeling like a victim may be affecting your food choices and weight.

Now go through every item on your list and ask yourself, "What is the smallest amount of accountability I can take to shift my experience toward something more desirable? Where can I 'eat a shit sandwich'?" In the right-hand column, write a sentence or two about how you can change your part in each dynamic. It might not feel pleasant to admit that you have contributed to a situation you are not happy with, but by taking some responsibility, setting better boundaries, or changing the way you view the situation, you will transform your role from victim to author. Now your story and, therefore, your life and weight loss are in your own hands.

PUNISHING STRATEGIES VS. PLEASURABLE STRATEGIES

A consistent pattern I've noticed in the women who are attracted to my work is that they have tried many of the diet books and methods out there. They come to me feeling profoundly cynical and jaded about weight loss, frequently saying, "Jena, you're my last resort." Though they can't always articulate exactly why other programs failed them, it's clear to me. The reason they feel hopeless is because unknowingly they've been pursuing what I refer to as the "punishing strategies" for weight loss. They haven't yet learned to become the authors of their lives, nor have they learned to trust the voice of the animal within. They are looking for an external solution.

The punishing strategies are the ones we've all tried with limited success. Whether it's Weight Watchers, Jenny Craig, no fat, low fat, no carb, high protein, or whatever the latest fad, these all encourage you to place your faith in the external power of "the expert" and neglect to empower the voice of your wise female animal. Whether they endorse calorie counting, nutrient restriction, counting points, or a daily weigh-in, punishing strategies encourage us to say no to our own instincts and to follow their rules. While it's possible to lose weight by restricting yourself, you will still be plagued by feelings of limitation, which is neither fun nor feminine.

For example, the deprivation approach to dieting is punishing because it is stressful. You beat yourself up if you can't stick to the program, and you feel worried and guilty every time you eat. My heart breaks when I meet a woman on a restrictive diet. There's always a look of pain and restraint in her eyes, as though she's stuck in a small cage guarded by calorie-counting and portion control. These women aren't honoring themselves; instead, they're acting aggressively toward their female animals. Time and time again, when diets fail, women blame themselves or feel victimized, not recognizing the lunacy of the punishing approach itself.

Another failure in the punishing approach is the excessive focus on numbers. Now I'm not trying to say that numbers unto themselves are bad. Garrett Gunderson, author of *Killing Sacred Cows,* puts numbers in perspective: "Numbers can be valuable tools when we place them in the right context, but when we overvalue them, they cloud our judgment and negatively influence our decisions. Numbers can be used to manipulate, overemphasize, and deceive." The truth is numbers are neutral, but the way we use them can be dangerous. If you allow the number on the scales to determine your self-worth, your level of happiness, or how good you deserve to feel today, you are making a big weight loss mistake. The trap of the punishing strategies is giving these numbers disproportionate relevance in your life.

I had been working with my client Judy for a few weeks, and she was making incredible progress. She was making different food choices, dressing differently, feeling better in her body, and had started swimming at a local pool. Then she checked her bathroom scale, and much to her dismay, she had gained a pound. This pound could easily have been composed of muscle, as muscle weighs more than fat, but in her mind the number on the scale told her she was a failure. She felt so bad about herself that she lost the momentum to continue with the healthy choices she had been putting in place. It took her weeks to get back into her groove.

To prevent you from making that same mistake, I recommend that you throw away your scales. There are other, better ways to judge your progress: how you feel in your body and how your clothes are fitting.

Numbers give us quantities, but what we are really trying to achieve is a quality. Aiming for a number on the scales or counting the calories that cross your lips is ultimately of no help. Aiming for a feeling that you want to experience is something useful to achieve. For example, if your goal is to weigh 150 pounds, what do you expect this 150 pounds to feel like? A number doesn't feel like anything! What you really want is to feel happy, sexy, sensual, and alive. What's more, your weight will never be a fixed number. Women's bodies are ever changing by nature, and it's completely normal to fluctuate up or down five pounds over the course of a month due to hormonal changes tied into your menstrual cycle.

While the punishing strategies can result in temporary weight loss, they do not address the qualities that you want to experience in your body nor the quality of your food or your life. Sure, some diets may contain kernels of useful information, but they highlight only one small piece of the weight loss puzzle. Punishing strategies limit your food options and can steer you toward "diet" foods, which aren't all that appealing or good for you, but are recommended because of their low caloric value. For example, a diet soda or a frozen diet entrée might seem to be a perfect choice according to the numbers-based punishing strategy, but does your female animal really enjoy either of these, and do they nourish her in the long run?

Most important, the punishing strategies are simply no fun. And because they're not enjoyable, the stress they cause prevents you from ever achieving the relaxation response we're meant to experience, which is why punishing strategies will always, over time, lead you to put back on the pounds you lost or, worse, lead to more weight gain.

For a woman to lose weight successfully, her methods need to be as feminine as she is. That's why I teach pleasurable strategies for weight loss. They allow women to slim down permanently in a way that restrictive dieting never can. The reason pleasure is such a great boost for weight loss is that it has the power to shift the mode of the body from stressed, anxious, or unaware to tuned in and turned on.

Even if you do succeed in losing weight with a punishing approach, it will feel like a punishment to maintain—and seriously, who wants to live like that? A pleasurable approach, on the other hand, creates a result that is a pleasure to maintain. With nothing to rebel against, the pleasurable approach is the secret to lasting results because it activates the relaxation response. Whereas the old-school approach is all about setting your eye on a goal and plotting the most direct and logical path to reach it, the pleasurable, feminine approach goes about it a different way. By focusing on achieving the end result—the pleasure of feeling great about your body—at the beginning, you won't need to pull out your calorie counter or spend even ten minutes on a treadmill if it doesn't bring you pleasure. The pleasurable strategies embrace numbers only when they are helpful (for example, when following a recipe).

Where the punishing strategies push and patrol your body, the pleasurable strategies awaken the genius inside of you. Your wise female animal already instinctively knows what to eat and how to move to be in shape. A pleasurable experience makes you feel light and buoyant. A punishing experience makes you feel heavy and bleh! Once you realize this, you'll see that punishing yourself to lose weight is insanity. Best of all, the pleasurable strategies allow you to eat the foods you love and to recognize when you are full and satisfied. There are no restrictions of any sort: you can literally have your cake and eat it, too! No food is forbidden as long as it gives you true pleasure. But your pleasure can change from bite to bite, so what you learn is to pay close attention to what lights you up in real time. This way you can continue to eat the foods you and your female animal love in the right amounts.

Punishing Weight Loss Paradigm	Pleasurable Weight Loss Paradigm
My body is an untrustworthy beast.	My body is a wise female animal.
My body is an "it."	My body is a "she."
My body is a possession I control.	My body is a creature I protect.
Pleasure with food is a bad thing.	Pleasure with food is a good thing.
Pleasure is an occasional reward.	Pleasure is a vital daily nutrient.
I can't eat what my body wants.	I can eat what my body wants.
Weight gain is a sign my body has failed.	Weight gain is my body's cry for attention.
Food is my body's enemy and foe.	Food is my body's friend and ally.
My appetite is too big.	My appetite is perfect.
An outside authority tells me what to eat.	My body knows what to eat.
Exercise is work for my body.	Exercise is play for my animal.
I'm ashamed of my body.	I'm proud of my body.

THE MOST PLEASURABLE THINGS ARE FREE

When you are able to feel fully, without reservation, you will be able to take advantage of the wonderful fact that though there are many sources of pleasure, the greatest pleasures (which are also labeled taboo) are free, or close to free—sexual pleasures, olfactory pleasures, and the pleasures of the palate. It's free to relish the feel of the breeze on your skin or to lie in a park and listen to the sound of the birds. It is free to touch yourself sexually or to be touched by someone else. Delicious fresh foods do not have to be expensive. As self-love expert Michel Madie told me, "The fact that accessing pleasure is a conscious choice and that the best ones are virtually free is the most extraordinary socialist principle of our human existence."

3 The Science of Pleasurable Weight Loss

WHEN I BEGAN to trust my body and trust pleasure as a way of life, the weight I had been holding onto began to melt away. Trusting my desires had catalyzed a profound shift in my body. I knew I was happier and more relaxed, but what I didn't know was that there was a real biological reason why finding my pleasure with food and life was helping me lose weight. Marc David, founder of the Institute for the Psychology of Eating, taught me how pleasure is directly related to the science of weight loss.

The scientific foundation for my approach to weight loss is the biochemistry of pleasure, a powerful metabolic catalyst that stimulates digestion, assimilation, and, you'll be thrilled to know, calorie burning. What typically makes weight loss so challenging, even for women who are used to success in other areas of life, is that our metabolism is ruled by two distinct collaborations between the mind and the body: the central nervous system (CNS) and the autonomic nervous system (ANS). Although you can consciously direct your hand to pick up a cup, you can't just tell your body to lose weight and expect her to obey. That's because, as its name implies, the ANS organizes the physical responses we can't consciously control. If you've ever been sexually aroused when you didn't intend to be, that's your ANS at work. Similarly, when you haven't been able to lose weight despite your attempts, it is also your ANS that is responsible.

The ANS is a barometer for our sense of safety or danger, and accordingly it engages one of two modes, the sympathetic or the parasympathetic nervous system. You can think of these like an on-off switch; you're either in one mode or the other. The one thing that controls your ANS response is how much stress you are experiencing and how you handle it when it occurs.

We all know that we experience stress from external cues (our job, our relationships, the weather, etc.). We also experience stress created by our state of mind (victim mentality, anxiety, bad self-esteem, or bad body image, etc.) or by physical changes in our body (pain, hormonal changes, etc.). What you might not know is that when we are under stress, our connection to our animal's wisdom is impaired or even silenced. But when we are completely relaxed, those lines of communication are wide open, and we hear her voice loud and clear.

My client Marjorie once told me she loves getting a professional foot massage. She said that while her feet are being rubbed, her animal speaks to her more clearly than at any other time. It's when she gets her body's biggest downloads of wisdom.

What's more, stress affects our metabolism, which affects our ability to lose weight. When we are in stress mode, the famous fight-or-flight response kicks in and activates the sympathetic nervous system. Despite the urban myth that stressing out about our weight is a necessary motivator for weight loss to occur, the biochemistry of the sympathetic nervous system actually causes the opposite effect. Once you understand the science behind this and take an honest look at all of the stressors you put yourself through in the name of weight loss, it becomes clear exactly why the overwhelming majority of people who lose weight on a diet gain it back within a year.

Signaling potential danger, the stress state makes survival the highest priority and instructs your body to protect itself through a host of biological responses. During the first two to four minutes of stress, your body burns through calories quickly, as you experience a rush of adrenaline. However, this increase ends abruptly, and when it does, metabolism slows down and becomes much less efficient—to the bane of stressed-out dieters everywhere. The body is encouraged to store weight in the face of stress rather than burn it off. This occurs as a cascade of reactions in the body, including a marked increase in the hormone cortisol and the brain chemicals adrenaline and noradrenaline, all of which hinder weight loss. Excess cortisol production corresponds to an increase in the production of insulin, the fat-storing hormone that is your body's most effective tool for preserving calories and storing them in the form of fat for later use. This fat formation typically occurs around the belly. Adrenaline and noradrenaline shut down digestive activity and redirect blood flow from the stomach to the brain (for fast thinking) and to the arms and legs (for fast fleeing or fighting), all to support your survival of a perceived threat. "Fleeing" behaviors are also demonstrated in forms of "avoidant coping," such as social withdrawal, compulsive eating, or substance abuse.

Another aspect of the stress state is a "freeze response." This is the classic deer-in-the-headlights reaction, where instead of fleeing or fighting, a creature under stress will stand completely still or play dead to confuse a predator so it will move on to another object of prey. If you feel stuck in your ways—whether it's a pattern of overeating or compulsive dieting, an unhealthy relationship, a job you hate, or even too much time zoning out in front of your TV or computer—chances are, you're caught in the freeze response. But you don't have to stay frozen forever. You can learn to release the stress that is keeping you stuck so that you can begin to create the life of your dreams.

The term *tend and befriend* describes another stress-related set of behaviors women often exhibit. This response refers to our unique instinct to protect our offspring (tending) and to come together in groups in threatening times (befriending). Women are rewarded for these behaviors with the release of the brain chemical oxytocin, known as the love hormone, which signals the good feeling we receive from nurturing others. But if you find yourself taking care of others when you really should be taking care of yourself, this is evidence that you are using the tend-and-befriend response to your disadvantage. Alternatively, you can learn to let the innate desire to tend and befriend come to your own aid instead of another's. In effect, you will be showering yourself with the love and compassion you are so practiced in giving to others. You will be bathing your brain in the beneficial juices of the relaxation response, which set the stage for pleasurable, easy weight loss.

IS YOUR STRESS REAL OR IMAGINED?

Your body does not distinguish between a real and an imagined threat. The thought of a threat in itself is enough to set off the stress response. Whatever the source, if you're stressed out, you're telling your female animal not to lose weight.

Gaining weight under stress actually helped our ancestors survive: the body understood that the bigger they were, the more protected they were. Extra weight meant they were better equipped to survive famine because they were bigger than the creature next to them, which meant not getting attacked and living longer.

Today, the same survival strategy that once helped our ancestors can now work against us if we try to lose weight in a stressed-out manner. The stress of our modern existence is already so pervasive that it's likely you've been pushing your animal too hard for too long. Many of us have been living in chronic stress, with little to no soothing or comfort, and we've gotten so used to it that we don't even know how stressed out we are.

I'm not saying that life must only be blue skies and daisies in order for you to lose weight; however, stress can be a temporary incident instead of a sustained way of life. It really is up to you to learn how to manage the stresses that are presented to you and to discard the ones you create for yourself. For example, when you feel stressed out from self-imposed food deprivation or you allow the negative self-talk of a bad body image to circulate unchecked in your mind, you are triggering the internal biochemistry that actually prevents the weight you wish to get rid of from dropping—no matter how successful you may be at restricting yourself.

If we are honest with ourselves, we will see that many of our stressors are the product of self-created narratives. They can be the incessant negative thoughts that play over and over in our minds or the endless shame we feel about our bodies. When this happens, we are signaling an alarm, and the brain responds with the stress response. The invisible thoughts in the privacy of our minds are undoing our best efforts, sending a signal to hold on to weight. Even if you can't admit you're participating in this cycle, you can't lie to your ANS, so you still pay the price.

Furthermore, as every dieter knows, dieting itself makes you feel uncomfortable, which prompts you to search for something that will ease your burden. Before you know it, your hand is back in the cookie jar, which leads to more guilt, more shame, and a renewed resolve to further restrict, control, and deprive yourself once again. The relentless cycle then continues.

The body's message is clear: any diet or exercise program that stresses you out is a doomed-to-fail strategy. Deprivation, dieting, self-judgment, guilt, shame, rules, regulations, regimens, points, charts, scales, plans, portion control, calorie counting, tedious treadmills, punishing exercise regimes, a no-pain-no-gain attitude—unless you are the rare bird who happens to enjoy them, all these approaches are stressful, which means it's scientifically sound to say that they are not going to work.

That's why I consider weight gain to be a woman's personal angel. Yes, you read that correctly—angel, not devil. As counter-intuitive as it may sound, weight gain is your angel because it delivers a sacred message that essentially says, "Whoa, girl! You are way too stressed out. Your misery has gone on for too long. You need to relax." When you realize this, you can begin to shift your attitude. Instead of thinking, "Weight gain is happening *to* me," you understand, "Weight gain is happening *for* me to learn and grow."

Your Pleasurable Weight Loss challenge is to embrace the hidden message in your weight gain. For as much as you may loathe your shape and abhor your relationship with food, it has succeeded in drawing your attention to what you had otherwise been neglecting. Through weight gain and food compulsions, your female animal is succeeding in getting your attention to let you know she's not happy.

The good news (which I hope will give you a sigh of relief) is that the cure for all your stress is the relaxation response. This phenomenon has long been understood by Eastern healing and wisdom traditions and was more recently identified in the West by Dr. Herbert Benson in 1975. Here's how it goes. When you are relaxed, your parasympathetic nervous system is dominant, and your body receives the message that life is safe. Liberated from the need to protect against danger, your body is primed to "rest and digest," which means letting go of the extra weight it stored for protection. Your digestion and assimilation are optimized, calorie-burning efficiency is heightened, and your body's ability to communicate fullness and satisfaction to your brain after you've eaten is enhanced. When you are relaxed, your entire system is wired to lighten up—physically, mentally, and emotionally. This is the ideal condition for losing weight.

Even the least tech-savvy person knows that when your computer is acting up, you turn it off, let it rest for a moment, and then reboot, and more often than not, that solves the problem. The relaxation response has the same effect on your body. It's your own system reboot. Also known as the regenerative mode and the rejuvenation mode, the metabolic state of relaxation is when healing occurs. When you feel like you're coming down with something, go to bed, and wake up in the morning feeling like a new person, you've rebooted during your hours of sleep. You allowed your body to enter a relaxation state, and your immune system was able to do its job. The secret to lasting weight loss is to shift your nervous system from chronic stress to a consistent relaxed state.

My client Rosa led a very busy life. She was a nurse at a big-city hospital, as well as a wife and mother. She was so accustomed to giving her energy and attention to others that taking time out to do something purely for herself never even occurred to her. It was only when she came to me to address her weight gain that she learned the connection between relaxation and metabolism. At my urging, she became willing to make taking time to chill out a priority. I suggested that Rosa break the cycle of her chronic stress by reserving thirty minutes a day to do anything she found relaxing. Rosa enthusiastically committed to the practice. During this time, which she came to call her "half-hour of power," sometimes she sang, sometimes she stretched or danced, and sometimes she closed her eyes and daydreamed. I also suggested she stay away from the computer during this time dedicated to pleasure. Rosa later told me that those thirty minutes a day were making a world of difference in reducing her overall stress levels and that her body was feeling slimmer and lighter already.

Stress Mode	Relaxation Mode
Sympathetic nervous system dominance	Parasympathetic nervous system dominance
Fight-or-flight-or-freeze mode	Rest-and-digest mode
Focus on surviving	Focus on thriving
Cortisol increases	Cortisol decreases
Insulin increases	Insulin decreases
Fat storage increases	Fat burning increases

WHAT PLEASURE HAS TO DO WITH IT

When your life includes ample pleasure, not only will you lose weight effortlessly, but your life will also be much more fun. Pleasure triggers relaxation, and relaxation triggers weight loss: anything that helps you relax is going to support your animal to let go of her excess weight.

One of the myths about pleasure is that it must be an over-the-top, decadent, or extravagant experience. But it's the simple pleasures that are often the most gratifying. They are also readily available to you on a daily basis. No matter how simple or complex, though, all types of pleasure will help to put you in the relaxation state. Some of my favorite stress-releasing, relaxation-promoting activities include the following, and you can add your own:

- Dancing
- Singing
- Listening to or playing music
- Being in nature
- Laughing
- Taking a hot bath or shower
- Having an orgasm (more on that in Chapter 7)
- Engaging in arts, crafts, or other creative pursuits
- Playing
- Giving yourself time to do nothing

There are also three distinct practices that can immediately reduce stress: deep breathing, quality sleep, and meditation.

RELAXATION BEGINS WITH THE BREATH

Conscious breathing is the most potent way to soothe both body and mind, and it has the power to shift your metabolism to the pleasurable weight loss mode. With just three deep breaths, you can literally change your physiology from the stress state to one of complete relaxation, thereby dramatically altering your body's baseline calorie-burning ability. Even if you are eating the healthiest food in the world, in ideal proportions, without learning how to breathe consciously, you cannot relax and, therefore, cannot stimulate weight loss. The reason is clear: you need to relax to lose weight, and you need to breathe deeply to relax. If you can learn to change your breath, you can learn to change anything about yourself, including your relationship with food, your weight, and your sense of self.

Stressed breathing is shallow, while relaxed breathing is rhythmic and deep. Breathe as slowly and as deeply as possible, right down to your belly, so that it puffs out when you inhale and contracts when you exhale. Take five to ten deep breaths. You can think of these slow, conscious breaths as a gift for both your body and mind, as each thrive in a relaxed state. You can practice conscious breathing with your animal while sitting, singing, meditating, chanting, eating, in movement (for example, during yoga, tai chi, or dance), as well as during sensual and sexual play.

PLEASURE PRACTICE
Letting the Mind Rest

The ultimate relaxation exercise in yoga is known as the corpse pose. Lie on your back on the floor or ground, with your palms facing upward, and let go of your thoughts. Bring your attention to your breath. Inhale through your nose and fill your belly, then your chest, and then your shoulders, with air. Exhale through your nose as well, releasing the air first from your shoulders, then from your chest, and then your belly. This breathing technique is called complete breathing, and it will help you to let your mind rest and release stress so that you can be in touch with the deeper wisdom of your female animal.

PLEASURABLE EATING PRACTICE 3
Relax Before You Eat

Just as fire needs oxygen to burn, your body requires a steady source of oxygen—which you provide through deep breathing—to maximize its calorie-burning efficiency. In just one or two minutes, deep breathing can significantly increase your oxygen intake and ignite your metabolism. Whenever you prepare to eat, first take several deep, conscious breaths to relax your body and mind and to prime your digestive fire with oxygen. Make sure you're sitting down, and pay attention to your posture, sitting with your weight distributed equally between both sides of your body, not slumping off to one side. Sitting in an uncomfortable position will only add to your stress, whereas sitting evenly and comfortably will lay the foundation for your whole physiology to come into a relaxed state in which your animal functions at her best. Close your eyes for a few seconds and simply concentrate on your breath until you can feel the stress or anxiety in your body or mind melt away. We don't want to channel stress or anxiety into how we eat. Chronic stress lowers your ability to experience pleasure, so you need to eat more to fill your biological pleasure requirement and feel satisfied. But eating when you are relaxed has the opposite effect: you reap more satisfaction from eating less.

THE PLEASURE OF A GOOD NIGHT'S SLEEP

One common way we neglect our animal is by depriving her of sleep. In a mind-oriented culture, it's easy to disregard the importance of sleep and to feel that what really matters happens while we're awake. For example, one of the big myths about weight loss that keeps women obsessed with intense workouts they don't enjoy is the mistaken belief that they're losing weight during high-impact exercise. The truth is that even though we do burn calories during exercise, the pounds don't come off until we're resting. What matters most for sustainable weight loss is how your body functions at rest, not how she functions in exertion.

Your animal needs her rest. It's crucial to make sure you get a good night's sleep because that's when your body heals and muscle grows. Although your mind may resist surrendering to the pillow, sleep will always be one of your animal's favorite activities. Frankly, I find nothing more relaxing than a good night's sleep. Sleep is one of the secrets of pleasurable weight loss. You may never be able to lose the weight you want if you deny yourself this simple pleasure.

When you don't get enough sleep, you become irritable and have a harder time the following day. When this happens, you are vulnerable to missing your animal's cues, which can lead you to make poor food choices in an effort to find foods that provide energy. An overtired brain is a hungrier brain. If you are constantly tired, you're more likely to overeat. Poor sleep also causes cortisol levels to increase, which signal your body to store fat and increase your overall stress level. Sleep, on the other hand, is one way to move from a chronic stress response to a relaxation response, making sleep one of the best ways to mitigate stress. As the Dalai Lama says, "Sleep is the best meditation."

Ideally, aim for eight hours of sleep each night. If you regularly wake up feeling tired, your animal is trying to tell you that you need to experience quality sleep more often. Create a pleasurable sleep ritual so that you wind down consciously and establish the best conditions for a good night's rest. When you go to sleep, keep the room pitch black. Consider moving your smartphone away from the bedroom so that you aren't tempted to keep your mind engaged when your animal really needs to sleep. Also avoid eating right before bed.

The pleasure of sleep is undeniable, but many women consciously sacrifice this pleasure in favor of "productivity." Don't cheat your animal of this necessary pleasure.

Let your animal take a catnap. Steal away for as little as twenty minutes during the day to lie down, close your eyes, and completely relax, guilt free. Whether you fall asleep or simply fall into a deep state of relaxation, remember that napping is another pleasure that is easy and free.

EATING WITH AWARENESS ACTIVATES PLEASURABLE WEIGHT LOSS

As Marc David teaches in *The Slow Down Diet,* when we eat with complete awareness and attention to our food, our bodies respond in distinct ways. First, we activate a connection between the brain and the body known as the cephalic phase digestive response (CPDR). The word *cephalic* comes from the Latin root meaning "of the head," and it refers to the release of digestive enzymes from foods we enjoy and from pleasurable eating experiences. When we start salivating with anticipation for foods we see and smell, that's the CPDR doing its job, activating our bodies' most efficient digestive enzymes.

Researchers estimate that without the benefits of the CPDR, as much as 30 percent to 40 percent of the total digestive response to any meal is compromised. This means that when you forgo the pleasure of eating with your senses engaged, you also forgo fully metabolizing your food, causing the body to store excess calories as body fat, which ultimately leads to weight gain. This is another sign from nature that pleasure and good health are designed to go hand in hand.

Being present while we eat is also critical for the relaxation response. Whenever we create a stressful state—which includes depriving ourselves of food or following a restrictive diet—our brains release a chemical known as neuropeptide Y. Neuropeptide Y has several functions, including increasing appetite and promoting the storage of fat. If you are eating in a feeding frenzy, without experiencing pleasure from the smell, taste, and texture of the food, then neuropeptide Y recognizes that you have missed out and signals your brain to seek more food so that you have another opportunity for the sensory gratification your brain is hardwired to receive.

These two responses teach us that we cannot escape the biological imperative for pleasure. If we miss out on the sensory satisfaction of the experience, the body will rebel by generating more hunger. And if we wolf down our food or subject ourselves to deprivation, we trigger the stress response and compromise calorie-burning efficiency, as we shut off the ability to perceive satisfaction. However, when we pay attention to our meals and engage the gentle power of relaxation and pleasure, we provide our bodies with the optimal scenario for complete metabolism.

The chart below explains how pleasure directly affects appetite and relates to the chemistry I've just described. Every time you eat is an opportunity to receive from food the pleasure your body biologically requires. But you must be present to the pleasure to receive it. If you're stressed out, multitasking, or simply not paying attention, you will not be able to experience the same level of pleasure you would if you were present and fully receptive to feeling the sensations of eating. If you feel guilty about the fact that you're eating, your attention will be on the guilt and not the sensations in your mouth. Knowing it's missing out on something important, your body generates hormones that stimulate your appetite, causing you to search for more food so that you have another opportunity for pleasure. If again you eat without presence to the pleasure, the cycle will continue until your body creates "forced relaxation," in the form of a food coma, at which point you will finally stop eating. On the other hand, if you do make a point to feel the pleasure that is available to you when food passes your lips, you will activate an alternative metabolic pathway that is ideal for weight loss. Relaxed and pleasured eating helps you fully digest your food and lets you know when you're full, eliminating the need for you to practice appetite control. You don't have to control your appetite because you are able to eat just the right amount by listening and paying attention to your animal.

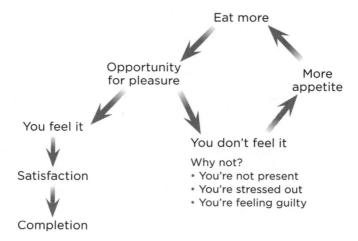

figure 2

I used to dream of a day when scientists would invent a "food pill" that would eradicate the need for eating altogether, but the CPDR and the actions of neuropeptide Y let us know that this day will never come. The science of metabolism shows us that eating is not just about taking in nutrients to keep the body working. For the body to optimally function, it also requires that eating is a pleasurable and satisfying experience.

When you are present to the pleasure of the food you eat, slowing down, relaxing, and enjoying every bite, you also activate a different metabolic pathway that is a great ally in pleasurable weight loss. Cholecystokinin (CCK) is a hormone released in the digestive tract that serves multiple functions. It stimulates the digestion of dietary fat and at the same time stimulates the pleasure sensors in the brain. It also sends a signal from the gut to the brain that lets you know when you've had enough to eat, effectively shutting down your appetite. If you've ever watched someone appear to be completely satisfied and leave food on her plate, chances are, that was CCK at work. So if you've feared that pleasure might cause you to overeat, CCK teaches us otherwise. CCK demonstrates how pleasure, appetite, and metabolism are beautifully and powerfully interconnected. Instead of trying to use willpower to control or suppress your appetite, being present to the pleasure of your meals will support your body in knowing naturally when she's had enough food. This very positive outcome depends on you being present.

THE PLEASURE OF MEDITATION

So often it feels like our thoughts are dominating our reality, drowning out the wise voice of our animals. Meditation is a practice intended to rest your mind by consciously focusing your attention inward, through your breath, a mantra, or visualization. By interrupting your cyclical thoughts, you recognize their transitory nature and that you are free at any moment to initiate a new thought.

Meditation improves concentration and helps us to be present, aware, and attentive in all aspects of our lives, including our eating and other pleasurable experiences. With practice, you'll be able to quiet your mind and find a centered, sacred space that you can return to whenever you are anxious or stressed. Meditation also triggers the relaxation response, allowing you to control your stress levels, reduce anxiety, and improve overall mood. Best of all, it teaches that you don't have to go outside of yourself to find pleasure. All you have to do to experience pleasure, or even ecstasy, is turn within.

Jon Kabat-Zinn, PhD, is well known for his research on meditation and has found that those who make it a regular practice become happier—which is why I consider meditation a true pleasure. People who meditate regularly report feeling "at one" or "connected" with the world. Whenever I meditate, I also experience a feeling of communion with the whole tapestry of existence.

PLEASURE PRACTICE
Meditation to Connect with Your Animal

Read through this exercise completely, and then you may want to record yourself reading the following meditation so that you can replay it during your practice. Or you could have a friend read it to you. Before you begin, place yourself in a comfortable and relaxing environment where you can completely let go of the stresses of your day.

Close your eyes and take a few deep breaths to relax. Visualize yourself lying in bed at night. Your eyes are heavy, and the bed is comfortable, soft, and warm. You are safe. As you drift off to sleep, notice how you intrinsically trust that your heart will keep beating all night long. You trust that even after you shut your eyes, in the morning you will be able to see again. You trust in your digestion and the multitude of other systems inside of you. In a state of deep trust, you relax into the pleasure of this bed, into the comfort of sleep, and into the release of letting go, knowing that in the morning, all of your parts will be here working.

Now imagine waking and entering your day with the same trust in weight loss. You trust that at the next meal, at breakfast, you will know what to eat, you will know when to drink, and you will know when to stop. You trust that you will remember to breathe as you eat, that you will know to chew as you eat, and that you will know how to slow down and savor every bite.

Now, continue through your day and visualize yourself trusting your body at lunch. Then see yourself eating your afternoon snack, feeling complete trust in your body. Now see yourself at dinner, trusting your hunger, trusting your appetite. You trust your female animal, the wise creature within you. You trust her to guide you exactly where you need to go to let go of excess weight that is not serving you.

See the happy smile on your face. Feel your female animal glowing from the inside, glowing because she's being acknowledged for who she is and the wisdom she carries. Notice how she thrives under relaxation and pleasure. Then, with one more deep breath, slowly come back to the present moment. Open your eyes, and carry the felt-sense of trust for your body with you into the day.

Give yourself some time to let the outside world disappear and take refuge in the pleasure of meditation. Prepare your space with soft pillows, candles, and incense, or meditate outside in nature. Discover the bliss within.

THE SECRET OF TRUST

When you trust your body, you can listen to what she says, and then let go and relax, which is when efficient calorie burning occurs. Now you may be thinking, "Trusting my body sounds like a great idea for other people, but not for me. When I listen to what she tells me to eat, I gain weight. I don't lose it." If so, your thinking is influenced by our culture, which has conditioned us to mistrust our bodies and the feminine in general. Learning to trust your body is a stance that needs to be reclaimed.

Instead of waiting for your body to earn your trust by conforming to your desire to lose weight on your terms, grant your body your trust now. Remember: she is the creature that keeps you alive. She is devoted to your well-being and deserves your trust. If her instincts seem untrustworthy to you, this is a sign to pay closer attention to what she is trying to communicate. You might find that what she is conveying, especially about food, is not what it appears to be on the surface. For example, if your animal is pointing you toward a candy bar, you can still trust that there's a reason. It may not be that you need sugar but a sign that you need something that candy bar signifies. You may need a snack, a full meal, a nap, or some fun and excitement.

Trusting your body is one way to show your love and devotion to your loyal life companion. Remember that it's when you are relaxed that you are most in touch with the trustworthy wise voice within. When you have full trust in your body, you will not only catalyze weight loss but also forge a more loving relationship with your animal—which is the foundation for a peaceful and pleasurable existence in every dimension of life.

Take care of your body. It's the only place you have to live.

JIM ROHN

4 Learning to Love Your Body

FOR MY CLIENT Cassandra, another day of waking up in her body equaled another day of self-loathing. Although we started to talk about the idea of loving her body, she protested that doing so at her current weight seemed delusional. "How could I possibly love my body at this size?" she rattled back at me. The world around her seemed to confirm that her body was unworthy of love and acceptance. From the media's messages that a woman's worth is dependent on her looking a certain way, to the echoes of her mother's negative comments since childhood about her body, Cassandra was convinced her body was inadequate. "I am not enough" was the deafening mantra she could not silence, no matter how hard she tried.

If Cassandra's story sounds familiar, it's because it describes the misery the majority of women feel about their bodies. That's why I refer to bad body image as the silent killer of weight loss; it is the unspoken thoughts that have the most power to sabotage us. Many of the women who feel shame, anger, and resentment about their "fat" bodies don't realize that their negative feelings can actually be causing them to gain weight and preventing them from losing it.

The statistics are horrifying. According to Margo Maine, PhD, author of *Body Wars: Making Peace with Women's Bodies,* 54 percent of 13-year-old girls feel unhappy with their bodies—a number that rises to 78 percent for 18-year-olds. From my anecdotal research, I'd say that number is closer to 95 percent. Some women would say they don't know a single woman who truly loves her body, without reservation. Tragically, there are even girls as young as five or six years old who describe themselves as "being on a diet."

When I was a teenager and first learned that the photos of gorgeous women in magazines are airbrushed, I naively didn't believe it. Nowadays, advertisers rarely release photos of women that haven't been digitally altered to make them look inhumanly perfect. A fashion photographer once described such images to me as "photo art," as opposed to actual photography. The result is that we end up comparing ourselves to standards of beauty that don't exist outside of Photoshop. No matter our size, we can never measure up to these unreal images. Caroline Heldman, PhD, a professor of politics who specializes in the media, makes a strong point: "This is the first time in human history that marketers have dictated our cultural norms and values." No wonder most women feel trapped in perpetual inadequacy.

Here in the United States, we are so conditioned to perceive the bodies of thin models and actresses as "normal" that even women with a healthy body size suffer from a distorted view of their bodies and experience a form of imagined ugliness. But it doesn't have to be this way. In other places around the world, women have a better body image. They haven't been conditioned to think their bodies fall short of perfection, so they appreciate a wide range of body sizes.

The billions of dollars spent every year to reinforce images of how we "should" look, in order to sell products and services that supposedly solve our problems, continue to remind us of how we fail to meet such beauty ideals. We've been trained to believe that if only we had the "perfect body," we would also have the "perfect life." (Just look how happy all these women seem, right?) But these images offer an illusion, a promise that is a bald-faced lie. I'm sure you've known plenty of thin women who can't stand their bodies or their lives. Being thin or gorgeous does not guarantee that you will have a dream life or that you will love yourself.

PLEASURE BITE

Adorn your animal with exquisite accessories that will make her feel beautiful. Earrings, scarves, bracelets, or a statement necklace don't have to be expensive to look fantastic, and they can provide a feeling of pleasure, femininity, and sensuality.

THE VICIOUS CYCLE OF BAD BODY IMAGE

While you might think that the reason you want to lose weight is simply because you don't like the shape of your body, this is an oversimplification. Deeper within yourself, you'll discover that behind your wish to look a certain way lies the desire to love your body and yourself—which is the most natural wish of all.

When you don't love your body, you are caught in the grip of a victim story. You facilitate the illusion that your body is causing you pain, and so you perceive yourself as the victim of your body's flaws and failings. Trapped in a self-obsession that consumes precious time and mental and emotional energy, you are held back from fully engaging in the things that can bring you pleasure, such as creativity, connecting with others, and making a difference in the world. When you give your bad body image significance, your negative self-involvement causes you to miss out on the deeper meaning of existence. This in turn motivates you to punish your body, victimizing your female animal and perpetuating the cycle of disconnection and disempowerment. Your bad body image is the ultimate betrayal of her and yourself. In effect, you are saying to her and yourself, "You're not good enough, and I'm ashamed of you."

When you don't love your body, you may want to hide from the world. Your fortress of self-disapproval might keep you isolated from others. I've heard so many tragic stories of women who decline invitations to parties, family gatherings, and once-in-a-lifetime opportunities because they don't want to be seen.

Do you want to go to the grave not loving your body? Imagine your loved ones standing next to your coffin, commiserating,

"What a shame! She never realized how beautiful she was. She loved other people but not herself." But you can change that and make a conscious choice to accept that you are being too hard on yourself. You've got to let go of your self-directed negativity right now, with me as your witness, and start loving yourself and your body, no matter your size.

One of the tools most of us have been unconsciously trained to use to fuel change is shame. As a child, when you did something you weren't supposed to do, your parent may have said, "Don't do that! You should be ashamed of yourself!" In this way, shame has become ingrained as our go-to emotion when we notice something about ourselves we don't like and want to change. Most women think negative self-talk about their bodies is harmless because it only happens inside their heads. What they don't know is the metabolic ripple effect their inner talk creates.

Let's look at bad body image from the perspective of your female animal. So there you are, looking in the mirror, saying all kinds of nasty, critical things about your body, thinking that no one can hear you because it's all in the privacy of your mind. But she hears every word! Every insult cuts her like a knife. She feels shamed and denigrated, and not surprisingly, this is a stressful experience for her. And remember: because stress triggers weight gain, your bad body image becomes a self-fulfilling prophecy. The weight gain that ensues is then used as justification for more self-loathing, and so what I call the Infinite Body-Shame Loop goes round and round.

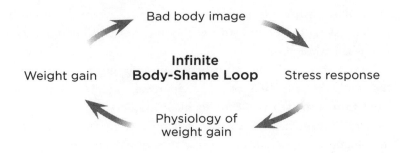

figure 3

Furthermore, when you are in the stress of the Body-Shame Loop, your connection to your body's wisdom is dulled, as is your sensitivity to pleasure, so your experience of life becomes more lackluster. This in turn likely causes you to eat even more in an attempt to make up for your desensitization to all pleasures, including food.

STOP WAITING TO LOVE YOURSELF BECAUSE OF YOUR WEIGHT

When you hate yourself and your body, you view pleasure as the enemy, and you deny yourself pleasure out of spite. You only have one life, and you can't afford to waste it hating yourself or denying yourself pleasure, even if you are in a body that is not magazine-perfect. I want you to wake up and be outraged that until now you have let extra weight on your belly and thighs jeopardize your opportunity to embrace the glory of being alive. If you had a child with a physical disability, would you love her any less? Of course not! So look beyond what you perceive as your body's physical imperfections and love her as profoundly and unconditionally as you would your own child.

As I learned from Marc David, although we think looking good will be the magic that finally makes us feel good about ourselves, the reality is the opposite: feeling good will make us think we look good. Have you ever noticed that your body image varies, even within the course of a day? Have you ever gotten dressed in the morning, thinking you looked terrible, but later something unexpectedly wonderful happened and your mood brightened? And you then started to think, while wearing the very same outfit, that you actually looked pretty good? Or think of when you are in the throes of sensual or sexual pleasure. There's no mental space available for you to start thinking you look bad because you're focused on a feeling rather than a conscious thought—you're focused on a feeling of pleasure. When you are engaged in the moment and feeling great, your attention is on your experience, and any thoughts of a bad body image cease to exist. In effect, you are crowding out the bad thoughts and replacing them with a positive feeling.

When you are in your pleasure, your mind surrenders, and you stop worrying. When you feel good, no longer listening to your inner verbal attack, your body also relaxes, and lo and behold, you have the experience of feeling you look good. As your attention shifts from how bad you look to how good you feel, over time, without even trying to lose weight, you will slim down—which in turn supports your good body image. Then you find yourself in a virtuous cycle I call the Infinite Body-Love Loop. In other words, pleasure, the heroine of our story, is yet again the catalyst that breaks the cycle.

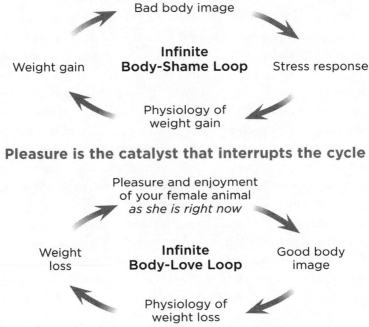

Bad body image

**Infinite
Body-Shame Loop**

Weight gain

Stress response

Physiology of
weight gain

Pleasure is the catalyst that interrupts the cycle

Pleasure and enjoyment
of your female animal
as she is right now

Weight
loss

**Infinite
Body-Love Loop**

Good body
image

Physiology of
weight loss

figure 4

If you are waiting until you think you look good to allow yourself to really experience pleasure and feel good, you'll be a dog forever chasing its tail. You can count on the mind to arrive at the conclusion that you are not good enough. So if you are waiting to think you look good in order to feel good, you may wait forever, no matter what you weigh.

To embark on the pleasurable journey of developing a positive body image, the most fundamental way to feel good is to feel good about being alive. Anyone can access this feeling at any time because it is simply a shift in awareness, from complacency to gratitude—regardless of your struggle with your weight and food.

Loving yourself is a wonderful and liberating feeling, and it is a requirement for receiving pleasure and fully authoring your life. When you love yourself, you have so much more energy, inspiration, and mental and emotional capacity to bring to the world and to create for yourself a life of true pleasure. If you're caught in a downward spiral of thinking that you need to lose weight to feel good about your body, it's time to wake up to the realization that you've been trying to win an unwinnable game. In the same way that the media has made being thin the answer to all your dreams, I'd like you instead to make loving yourself and your body the key to your dreams. Loving yourself is a gateway that just being thin can never be.

The Infinite Body-Shame Loop and the Infinite Body-Love Loop are mutually exclusive. You can't enjoy your body and be ashamed of it at the same time. Losing weight is not the ticket to loving your body, nor is it the ticket to experiencing pleasure in your body or your life. Unless you learn how to experience pleasure now, losing a dress size is not going to do it. No matter how you look, your female body can still be a source of tremendous pleasure. There's nothing your female animal wants more than that. And when you're fully in your pleasure, you can't help but love yourself!

DO I DESERVE PLEASURE?

Now that you know that pleasure and enjoyment of your body are the keys to releasing your bad body image and to stimulating your metabolism so you can lose weight, the question becomes, what is holding you back? What is preventing you from taking this strategy and embodying it to the fullest?

There might be several reasons. You might feel afraid or ashamed of pleasure, or you might think that you don't deserve it, wondering, "Who am I to be having it when so many people go without?" Women have been conditioned to pass over pleasure for hard work and to think that a meaningful contribution to the world must involve sacrifice. We've been taught to believe sacrifice is noble and pleasure is a wasteful indulgence. We've been conditioned to believe that we need to be in control and to perceive surrendering and letting go as both a sign of weakness and a risk of danger. As you examine what's standing in your way of experiencing more pleasure, remember that dismantling a lifetime of programming takes time. If you have been told that seeking pleasure is selfish and narcissistic, be compassionate with yourself and your animal in the process.

The truth is that true pleasure doesn't lead you down such paths. Pleasure expands your ability to feel, and as you feel more, you can better connect and empathize with others. In the act of surrendering to pleasure, you let go of your grasp for control and allow yourself to be held in the loving arms of Mother Earth. As your female animal opens up physically and emotionally through pleasure, you become more engaged with life, not more self-involved. Self-loathing is the root of self-involvement, not self-love.

While you may have thought that pleasure was something you had to achieve, a deeper understanding of pleasure shows that it is not the case. Pleasure is always present, available for you, whether or not you pay attention to it, simply waiting for you to wake up and notice. When you view pleasure this way, it becomes apparent that when you take pleasure, you are taking it at no one's expense. Life is experiencing pleasure through you, and your pleasure does not come with a cost, because it is a gift. That's why there is no question about having too much of it or if by taking your fill, there will be less available for someone else. There's an infinite amount of pleasure for everyone. All we need to do is be aware.

From this viewpoint, the frame of reference is no longer even about having pleasure but about being pleasure. When you are pleasure, you appreciate that your baseline state is pleasure. An easy way to demonstrate this is through the corpse pose practice (see Chapter 3). In corpse pose, the chatter of your thoughts subsides, and your attention comes to rest in the pure sensation of your body's baseline state of pleasure.

It's important to remember that you are not your thoughts, no matter how seductively your mind will try to convince you otherwise. An individual thought is only a fleeting phenomenon in the larger context of who you are. Don't give thoughts the power to talk you out of loving your body and trusting pleasure. Once you realize that you are not your thoughts, it is easier to choose not to give them your attention and instead to tap freely into the pleasure of your animal body.

I'm not saying that once you awaken to pleasure there will no longer be pain, heartbreak, or suffering. There always will be. But when you make a practice of looking for the good and can relax into your circumstances, even in moments of anguish, you'll be able to connect yourself to the bigger picture and see the wonder and beauty in your own humanity. You will be able to harness a new willingness to stay open to the full spectrum of the human experience. While we can't be in a relaxed state of pleasure at all times, because that's not how life goes, I do believe we can live in grace. I define grace as a state of unbroken remembrance and gratitude for the gift of being alive. In other words, no matter what is going on, when we can be connected with the gratitude of being alive, we have a direct line to a pleasurable feeling.

In order to lose weight and keep it off, you have to embrace your deservingness of pleasure—and that sense of deserving comes from self-love. The more you love yourself and your body, the easier it will be to shower your female animal with pleasure. Let go of the phrase *guilty pleasure;* erase it from your vocabulary. True pleasures are always innocent. It's not possible to have a body you adore if you feel ashamed of feeling good. When you realize that you deserve pleasure, you become a role model of dignity and self-love for others. This is a contribution. As spiritual teacher and author Marianne Williamson writes:

> Our deepest fear is not that we are inadequate. Our deepest fear is that we are powerful beyond measure. It is our light, not our darkness that most frightens us. We ask ourselves, Who am I to be brilliant, gorgeous, talented, fabulous? Actually, who are you not to be? You are a child of God. Your playing small does not serve the world. There is nothing enlightened about shrinking so that other people won't feel insecure around you. We are all meant to shine, as children do. We were born to make manifest the glory of God that is within us. It's not just in some of us; it's in everyone. And as we let our own light shine, we unconsciously

give other people permission to do the same. As we are liberated from our own fear, our presence automatically liberates others.

4 PLEASURABLE EATING PRACTICE 4
Smell the Food

One simple way to begin to allow yourself to experience pleasure is the experience of eating. Whenever you sit down to a meal, bring yourself to a relaxed state and take a moment to deeply smell your food. You can do this by taking either long, slow inhalations, or rapid sniffs, like an animal, or a combination of both. A wine connoisseur closes her eyes to focus her senses on the depth and subtlety of the smell. Do the same with your food. Allow the aroma of the meal to be a distinct aspect of the overall pleasure of your eating experience. Consciously smelling your food helps to activate efficient digestion, which of course supports pleasurable weight loss.

THE PLEASURE OF FORGIVENESS

When you discover that there was a positive intention behind your struggles with food, you have found another secret for shifting your metabolism. Now that you are clear about all the things you have felt ashamed of and understand that they were intended by a deeper part of your psyche to help you, you can stop beating yourself up for your past actions. You can take a step back from your self-loathing and say, "My overeating was actually intended to accomplish something useful for me."

Until you forgive yourself, your struggle with food will feel like a war. Whether an actual armed conflict or a metaphorical conflict, such as the "war on drugs," war is a physical and psychological device that dominates our ecology. When we are at war, nothing changes. The key to ending the war with your body and to finding lasting peace is to recognize the positive intention that caused the war in the first place.

Can you remember a time when you had a fight with a loved one and felt outraged or bitter, only to find out later that your disagreement was based on a misunderstanding? Suddenly, your anger and resentment disappeared. It is the same with your war on your body. When you discover the underlying positive intention of your eating behavior, you realize that your anger with your body was based on a misunderstanding, and all the disappointment and disgust you have felt can vanish in an instant. You are then able to forgive your animal and yourself, and the war ends.

Forgiveness, especially of yourself, is one of the secrets of pleasurable weight loss because it fosters relaxation. Without forgiveness, a chronic low-level stress response that keeps you heavy is active. When you forgive yourself, the subsequent relaxation response affects your metabolism, and your baseline calorie-burning efficiency is optimized.

PLEASURE PRACTICE
Forgive Your Animal

Bring to mind all the ways you've felt your animal has triggered choices that led you to overeat and gain weight. Now forgive her for every one of these, knowing that behind every craving and choice was a deeper positive intention for you to feel good. Create a forgiveness ritual in which you vindicate your body of every crime you've ever accused her of. Whenever you find yourself irritated with your body, return to this state of forgiveness as your first step to getting back on track and in sync with her.

CHOOSING TO LET GO OF SHAME

For every woman who is struggling with weight, every time she eats, tries on clothes, or looks in the mirror, her silent companion is shame. You might be so familiar with shame that you wonder whether you would be motivated to lose weight if you didn't have it. Many women think shame is a necessary and useful reminder to stay focused on losing weight, that it protects them from giving in to their compulsions. While this might sound logical, the truth is that shame never yields lasting results. Sustainable change is driven by inspiration, not shame.

Shame is another stressor, so it triggers the metabolic processes that cause the body to hold on to weight, which we explored earlier. On an emotional level, stress hurts your self-esteem, eroding your natural confidence and enthusiasm. Also, shame and love are mutually exclusive. Love, appreciation, and pleasure cannot live where shame exists. So telling yourself you will love your body and be done with shame once your body is fit is not an effective stratagem. What's needed is to start loving your body just the way it is now.

Stop playing the punishing shame game, which doesn't feel good or win you anything, and instead choose to appreciate yourself as you are now. This is the strategy that will reward you with a slim, healthy body, and more. Start loving your body by trusting that you have it within you to make good choices. From now on, trust your ability to make good choices with your female animal. She knows what to eat and how to live. You can trust that what feels right to her is indeed right. Your animal will always be there for you. Even if you make a mistake with a choice, no matter what direction the wind blows, your animal will still be there to guide you home to yourself. Everything you think will come from losing weight will be available when you love yourself first, and loving yourself begins now.

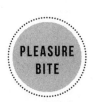

PLEASURE BITE

A song can change your mood in an instant. Check out the song "One Love" by Sara Tavares on her album *Balancê*. The lyrics say, "I need you, I love you, I can't live without you." As you listen to this song, put one hand on your heart and one hand on your belly and sing the words out loud to your beloved female animal, remembering that you need her, you love her, and you can't live without her.

THE POWER OF THREE SIMPLE WORDS

I was once at an event called Awesomeness Fest, where I listened to Broadway composer Jeff Marx tell a story about his friend Reese Rahman and their conversation about self-love. Reese had asked Jeff, "Can you look yourself in the mirror and honestly tell yourself 'I love you'?"

"I answered no, because like in a relationship, I wouldn't want to say it unless I meant it," Jeff told the audience. He then called an unsuspecting Reese up to the stage and handed him the microphone with these words, "Tell them what you told me."

Reese went on to tell his story: "I was feeling unsure of my path in life when I came across a book by motivational author Louise Hay, who recommends creating a practice of frequently telling yourself, 'I love you.' To make it more interesting than simply repeating the words over and over, she suggests turning it into a jingle. So there I was, in the shower, when all of a sudden, the melody came to me."

Reese started singing these words, "I love myself, I love myself, I love myself," and at the event, a packed room of three hundred people started singing along with him. The energy of the space exploded. The song was such a hit that even after the event, when all of us were home in our respective countries, we started making videos of ourselves singing "I love myself." Soon Reese's inbox was flooded with videos—so many that he created a website to share them, www.ilovemyselfsong.com.

PLEASURE PRACTICE
Tell Yourself "I Love You"

Saying "I love you" to yourself might sound corny, but there is something deeply profound about saying or singing those words to yourself. You can listen to Reese's version at www.ilovemyselfsong.com, or you can make up your own. I once had a client who realized that she told everyone she cared about that she loved them, except herself. She then began a practice each time she got in her car of taking a moment to put her hands on her heart and sincerely telling herself, "I love you."

Your turn. Take on this practice of verbally expressing your love for yourself on a daily basis. It's amazing what three words can do.

LOVE YOURSELF AND CHANGE THE WORLD
Now that you know feeling good is a necessary part of looking good, ask yourself, "Do I love myself enough to commit to feeling good?" Self-love expert Ariel White says, "As painful as hating

our bodies is, it is less scary than loving ourselves and opening ourselves up to the things that really, really matter to us." In other words, once you allow yourself to discover and embrace how beautiful, amazing, and powerful you really are, then not only will your personal world change but also you will free yourself up to change the world we share. In this way, the courage to love yourself is an act of activism.

Women are always beautiful.

VILLE VALO

5 The Feminine Principle

WE EACH POSSESS a combination of feminine and masculine energies. To lose weight, it is essential for women to contact our feminine side because it is the feminine principle that bestows the capacity to experience life through the body rather than the mind. I now consider myself a messenger for the feminine values that have been rejected and disowned by our male-oriented culture, but I didn't always understand the importance of feminine energy. Ironically, it wasn't until I read a book written to teach men the value of the feminine that I realized I needed to value the feminine within myself.

As I read the descriptions of the attributes of the masculine and the feminine, I was surprised to see that I related more closely with the masculine principles than with the feminine. At the time, I prioritized my business over my relationships, working long hours, and sometimes even slept on the couch in my office, instead of taking time to go home. I dressed in utilitarian black and felt lonely and isolated from other women. Nourishing my feminine side never made it on my to-do list.

Because our culture is so lopsided toward the masculine, women are starved of the joyous embodiment of the feminine. Many feel dried up emotionally and sexually and burnt out physically. When we are overly connected with the masculine, our energy flows up to our head rather than down to our hips, which causes upper-body tension and a diminished desire for sex and pleasure. Also, instead of dealing with tension as a feminine being would—with singing or dancing, for example—we respond with masculine coping mechanisms, like watching TV or drinking. When I realized how disconnected I was from my feminine nature, I knew that embracing it would be key to getting to the root of my food compulsion.

YOUR FEMININE LEGACY

The stereotype of women being the weaker sex is not in fact supported by evidence from the present or the past. When we look back at how humanity developed, the feminine has played a starring role. Women banded together and used their intuition to take care of the needs of the tribe. Long before there were hospitals, generations of midwives delivered babies; wise women were also healers, using plants, foods, and touch, among other modalities. Religion centered on the worship of the earth as a sacred mother. Nowadays, however, our feminine intuition is not a skill we are encouraged to develop. Instead, we are conditioned to ignore our intuition and to favor our masculine ability to reason.

But our intuition is the voice of our female animal, and the more we respect and listen to her wise guidance, the more we will get. As Annie Lalla told me, "Your masculine energy is the linear, problem-solving doer in you, while your feminine energy is your intuition and body wisdom. She's the visionary side of you, who is forever imagining what else might be possible. Your feminine side conceives ideas, while the masculine makes them so."

Indigenous cultures around the world still worship feminine energy, and you can, too. You can honor the force of the feminine by discovering and worshiping your own feminine energy. You don't need to look to the past to know what to do because you're at the front of the line: every woman is an evolutionary advancement of the women who came before her. Rejoice in the incredible gift and privilege it is to be a woman, and celebrate your feminine heritage.

Feminine energy fuels collaboration, kindness, tenderness, empathy, compassion, and receptivity. It is an orientation toward color, texture, taste, and all things sensual and sexual. When you cherish your feminine energy, you will cultivate a better relationship with your body, with food, and with pleasure, because the primary feminine value is that all life is sacred. This includes your body as it is right now!

Relationship expert David Deida teaches that the essence of the masculine is consciousness and the essence of the feminine is light. One of the qualities of the feminine is what is called *feminine radiance*. It is our power to radiate light from within. Light is the energy that radiates from the heart, and its nature mandates that it be seen. Being noticed and appreciated is one of the highest feminine values. Being seen makes women feel whole and loved. Girls dressing up in sparkly fairy wings are seeking the expression of their light and the feminine desire to be seen. This is why it is so debilitating for a woman to be unhappy with her body. When she feels unattractive, she will hide herself away, and when she is alone in this way, her self-esteem withers. She lacks the vital nourishment her feminine nature requires. But when women embrace their feminine radiance, we can contribute our light to any situation and brighten the mood for everyone.

Paying attention to my feminine side changed my life. For the first time, I gave myself permission to let my light shine without shame. I improved my posture and changed the way I dressed, favoring colorful, sensual, and playfully expressive clothes. I started spending money on things that bring me pleasure instead of saving all of my money for the abstraction of retirement. I dedicated a portion of my resources to enjoying my life now. At first I treated myself to little pleasures, like upgrading my hair conditioner to a fragrant organic one instead of the cheapest, most basic one. I purchased higher-quality foods, and I finally gave in to my desire to participate in a weekly salsa party near my office. I had wanted to attend for some time, but most weeks I pushed my desire to the side, prioritizing for working late and saving the ten-dollar cover charge for something more serious. Ten years later, salsa dancing

continues to bless me with pleasure. Imagine what you will discover when you embrace your feminine desires and values.

PLEASURE PRACTICE
Let Your Feminine Radiance Shine

Feminine radiance comes from the heart and can be mag-
nified by the face. Sharing your feminine radiance is a skill
that can be cultivated, and as you do, it can literally make
you look younger and more beautiful. One of the easiest
ways to increase your radiance is to soften the muscles in
your face. Intentionally relaxing and softening your face
helps you relax and shine your light. When you have a
soft face, you express receptivity to the world. People feel
invited to connect with you. If you would like to have
more relationships or closer relationships, a soft face is a
great asset. The softer and more relaxed you are, the more
open you are. Plus, soft lips make you very attractive to kiss.

Bring your awareness to the different parts of your face,
part by part. Soften your eyes, soften your jaw, and soften
your lips. Notice how much your entire body relaxes when
your face does. You can literally reduce tension in the mind
by softening your face. I've noticed my anxiety levels drop
as I have learned to relax my jaw.

CULTIVATING THE ART OF RECEIVING

While the punishing strategies suggest that you're going to lose
weight by *doing*—being more active, restricting your diet, changing
your habits—the pleasurable approach emphasizes cultivating the
feminine principle of *receiving* as one of its secrets. Mastering the art
of receiving is essential, as you can only experience pleasure to the
degree that you are willing and able to receive it.

We already know that when you experience pleasure, you put
your body into the relaxation state in which you burn calories
most efficiently and can effortlessly lose weight. Your ability to
receive therefore regulates the amount and quality of pleasure
you can enjoy and therefore the depth of relaxation you can attain.
To receive is to trust others, which puts you in the relaxation

state. When you are receiving, you are fully in your animal. Your mind becomes quiet and you stop making mental judgments. You interrupt stress, anxiety, and the cortisol response. You let go of expectations and control, and you surrender. This is why receiving is such an important skill to develop: it is literally the gateway to pleasurable weight loss.

Contrary to what most women think, receiving isn't passive. Like pleasure, when you are open to receiving you are present to your senses and aware of your desires. Instead of denying yourself, or subconsciously pushing away the gifts life seeks to bestow upon you, you are able to open yourself up to receiving them—whether they are compliments, opportunities, money, sexual attention, or simply the enjoyment of food or any other sensory pleasure.

There are two parts to learning how to receive. The first is to be more open and present to new sensations and experiences. The second is learning to ask for what you desire without commanding or ordering, but giving someone the choice to accept or decline without you being offended by their response.

In order to master the art of receiving, you first need to get clear on the hidden objections you may have. "Some women are intuitively good at receiving and some of us have to learn it," embodiment expert LiYana Silver told me. Culturally, women are conditioned to be good at giving and providing, but may feel ashamed or embarrassed about receiving, and therefore have never put attention to developing it as a skill. Women may feel vulnerable or powerless when they are invited to receive; they feel more in control when they are giving. Where this becomes an obstacle for weight loss is when you are only focused on giving, you are vulnerable to unconsciously turning to food because is it an easy, safe way to receive.

You may worry that by receiving, you will be indebted or obligated to someone else. While you may feel the pull to instinctively reciprocate, powerful receiving is an act that also rewards the one who gives. There is no greater example of this than in sex—giving to someone who is fully receiving is an ecstatic act of joy. You want to keep giving because you also feel like you are receiving. Allow yourself to receive without fixating on what you have to give back.

Another obstacle to receiving is a discomfort with the word "no," both in saying it and hearing it. When you have difficulty expressing boundaries, you may push away all new experiences and opportunities in a blanketing way rather than selectively receiving based on your authentic desires. The ability to receive depends on your discrimination about what comes in and what doesn't. You don't have to receive everything that is offered to you. Receiving requires honesty: don't say yes to please another. What's more, be willing to receive a "no" without interpreting it as a personal rejection.

You may feel that you don't deserve to receive until you lose weight. This belief will leave you feeling empty and cause you to overeat. If you make receiving conditional upon achieving a specific goal, like weight loss, then you'll always be postponing it and you'll find yourself in a never-ending cycle. To break this loop, examine the absurdity of the questions, "Who is to judge whether I am good enough to receive?" "What standards define my right to receive?" In reality, there is no judge and there are no standards. As my friend Ilan Kafri told me, "Just as you deserve to breathe because it's your birthright, it is also your birthright to receive."

The truth is, a woman's body is designed to receive. This can be sensually, sexually, physically, or emotionally. As LiYana Silver told me, "The feminine has an infinite capacity to receive." Instead of making your struggle with weight a reason you don't deserve to receive, interpret it as a reason to practice receiving all the more.

PLEASURE BITE

Let your feminine radiance be seen. Adorn yourself with clothes, jewelry, or makeup that shine or sparkle and bring out the light within you. This might be as simple as brushing a bit of glitter on your face or décolleté or wearing a sequined top, dress, or accessory.

THE FEMININE GIFT OF FEELING

The heart of the feminine principle is feeling. Women have a heightened capacity to feel, and one of the secrets of pleasurable weight loss is developing a willingness to make space for all of our emotions. Otherwise, we find ways to numb ourselves from the negative feelings we can't handle, and one of our most effective numbing strategies—you guessed it—is overeating. When you are willing to feel whatever emotion is present—whether it is anger, jealousy, or sadness—you don't need to take refuge in food to stuff down the unwelcome emotion. Whatever feeling you experience is an acceptable feeling to have. When you start nurturing your relationship with your feelings, it will ripple through every area of your life. You'll also be more attuned to your animal's messages.

I was raised to believe that there are "good" feelings and "bad" feelings and that the "good" ones are to be showcased while the "bad" ones need to be hidden. I spent decades trying to come across as confident, happy, generous, or any other "good" or "light" quality, and I wanted to hide all the ways I was scared, angry, and ashamed. Every time a dark emotion came up, I would immediately contract away from feeling it and cover it with shame, which made me feel horrible. Not wanting to have those dark feelings, I would turn to food and overeat, trying to change my state and make them go away.

The aspects of ourselves that we prefer to conceal from others make up what is known as our shadow. A classic way to spot your shadow is through your judgments of others. For example, if your sexuality is in your shadow, you will be critical or threatened by women who embody the full range of their sexuality. Another easy way to identify what is in your shadow is to look at what you judge in your mother. If you judge her for being impatient, unkind, or insensitive, those are the parts of yourself you are uncomfortable with.

I learned the lesson of appreciating the shadow side of myself from spiritual teacher Javier Regueiro. He once asked me, "Why only love 50 percent of yourself when you can love 100 percent?" Following his suggestion, I became committed to loving 100 percent of myself, my light side and my dark side. As I allowed myself to love and honor all of me, the energy I had been using to deny the darker parts of myself was liberated, and I felt an incredible, effervescent joy. Embodiment expert Amy Dawn Verebay told me, "When you deny your shadow, you are vulnerable to unconsciously overidentifying with the shame you are trying desperately not to feel."

HOW DO YOU WANT TO FEEL?

Many of us are not conscious that when we are aiming for a specific goal, what we are really looking for in that goal is the feeling we will experience when we attain it. For example, you might be set on losing a certain number of pounds, but what your female animal truly wants is the feeling you believe you'll have when you get there. As I said earlier, a number on the scale doesn't feel like anything, but you can define how you want to feel by other means. What you'd like to feel when you lose weight might include feeling sensual, light, feminine, sexy, peaceful, energetic, ecstatic, among a myriad of feelings. Having this level of clarity about how you want to feel is another secret of pleasurable weight loss.

Danielle LaPorte says in her book *The Desire Map*, "Knowing how you actually want to feel is the most potent form of clarity that you can have." When you are consciously aware of the feelings you desire, they operate as a guidance system. Your animal will let you know if you are going in the right direction. You flip a switch from judging yourself with the mind to feeling your experience in the body. If you are going in the right direction, the pursuit of the feeling becomes satisfying. This is another reason punishing strategies aren't effective in the long term and why focusing on how you want to feel is the better method. If you are enjoying the pursuit of your goals, you are more likely to be highly motivated to stay on the path.

For example, my client Serena told me that she wanted to lose thirty pounds. She also told me that she was frequently tired and believed that losing weight would make her feel energized. So, instead of focusing on the thirty-pound goal, I focused my coaching on her desire to feel more energized. I asked her to identify what foods, activities, people, and places made her feel more energized and to include them regularly in her life. Serena allowed herself to be guided by the desired feeling and began by giving herself permission to take short walks in the fresh air, drink more water, and decline social commitments that drained her. She noticed that sugary foods actually made her feel tired, so she was able to ease off her mid-afternoon sugar habit until it was completely gone. When she focused on attaining the energetic feeling, instead of losing thirty pounds, it became even easier for Serena to make good food choices throughout the day, and she never felt like she was punishing or denying herself because she had the experience in real time of how much better she was feeling.

Deeply inquire as to how you want to feel when you lose weight. Make an exhaustive list of all the ways you want to feel and identify your top five. Then let the pursuit of those five desired feelings guide your pleasurable weight loss.

FINDING YOUR PLEASURE THRESHOLD

Feelings can also be uncomfortable. You surely know about your pain threshold: the amount of pain you can sustain until it becomes too much to handle and your body tips into fight-or-flight metabolism. Along with a pain threshold, you also have a pleasure threshold. Most people don't realize that feeling pleasure is a skill to be cultivated. For example, if a new pleasurable experience generates more sensation than you are familiar with, this unknown feeling might be frightening.

Your ancient reptilian brain is responsible for coding every experience as either safe or unsafe. Every experience that hasn't killed you is considered not only survivable but also "safe" and, therefore, safe to be repeated—even if it was a dysfunctional or traumatic experience. Anything unknown is coded as "unsafe." That's why you might feel scared and nervous or hold yourself back when you are experiencing greater heights of pleasure than you've previously known. Even if your mind expects that something "should" be pleasurable, like a romantic date, that it is unknown causes your reptilian brain to respond with alarm bells in an effort to save you: "No way! Don't go there! You are outside your safety zone!"

In response to the reptilian brain's reaction, your mammalian brain interprets the experience with fear, anxiety and skepticism, while the neocortex makes sense of the feelings by creating a justification for the reptilian brain's reaction. You'll find yourself coming up with rationalizations that explain why you shouldn't be having this much pleasure, which can easily land you right back in a stress response, which we know promotes weight gain, which is what you were seeking pleasure to escape! What happens here is that you hit your pleasure threshold, which triggered the fight-or-flight response instructing you to avoid the experience.

Annie Lalla says that when you hit your pleasure threshold you will avoid the experience by redirecting your attention to any possible distraction that lessens the intensity of the sensation in your body. But this response also prevents you from fully relaxing into the sensation. For example, if you're on the verge of experiencing more sexual pleasure than you've previously known, you might find yourself suddenly thinking about your to-do list. If you continue to limit yourself to the existing parameters of your nervous system, you may find yourself sentenced to a life with food as your principal source of pleasure.

Your present-day calibration of what is safe, which influences these responses, was first imprinted when you were a child. As a little one, when a sensation became too much for you to handle, you withdrew your attention from the sensations in your body and sought refuge in a narrative in your mind. For example, shouting in the house that was too much for your young nervous system to handle could have caused you to disassociate from your body to the safety of your imagination. While this avoidance strategy helped you survive when you were four, it no longer serves you as an adult. When you retreat into your thoughts, you also abandon your female animal.

While you've already identified some reliable sources of pleasure, the pursuit of discovering something new is always alluring, and because new pleasurable experience will create intense sensations in the body, you need to be ready for them. If you want to be free to author your life and to have more pleasure than ever before, you are bound to confront the edge of your own ability to consciously hold sensation in your body. So you must develop skills that will allow you to go beyond your current pleasure threshold.

The way to expand your pleasure threshold is to learn to turn off the brain's alarm bells and to recalibrate your nervous system so that your ability to receive and sustain pleasure increases. Activating this capacity is one of the secrets of pleasurable weight loss because your response to pleasant sensation has the power to shift your metabolism from the stress state to the relaxation state. Transcending your current pleasure threshold requires deep reprogramming, over time and with awareness. But with a true desire to feel more, you can rewire your nervous system to extend your pleasure threshold. As you begin to feel more, you will experience your animal's delight, essentially saying to you, "I want to feel. I was born to feel. How can we live like this all the time?" Such growth and transformation will allow you to gift your body with pleasure and to let your female animal know just how much she is loved and rewarded by you.

LIFTING THE PLEASURE THRESHOLD
BEGINS WITH A RETURN TO RELAXATION

Before you advance to feeling more pleasure, you first need to establish a fundamental feeling of safety. This is another way of describing the relaxation state. If you are numb from stress and then try to add pleasurable sensation to your system, it won't be a true pleasure because you won't be able to fully feel it. It is nearly impossible to feel resistant and unsafe with a new pleasure and to relax into it at the same time. This is why we have to take a step back to create a baseline relaxation state first, which will be your foundation for true pleasure.

The tool for doing this is called self-regulation, crucial for weight loss and actually for most anything in life. Self-regulation is largely achieved by being present. According to early-parenting expert Cecily Miller, "Self-regulation is a powerful invitation to build your capacity to stay present with yourself and to love and honor yourself enough to make staying present in your body, behind your eyes, and in your belly, a high priority."

Though women value our ability to please and attend to others, in reality, learning to stay present first with ourselves, with our physical and emotional needs, is of more value to the world. Yoga, meditation, tai chi, and other awareness-based practices help us develop the skill of self-regulation, of moment-to-moment presence. By making self-regulation part of your daily practice and taking care of yourself first, you will also be taking care of your animal and supporting your weight loss.

To embrace self-regulation is to embrace true adulthood, for you alone are responsible for your state of being—no one else is coming to save the day. If food makes you feel safe and comforted, it makes sense that you have been turning to food when you need soothing. But when you equip yourself with the tools of self-regulation, you will be able to bring your nervous system back to a calm, relaxed state. You'll find that you no longer have to use food to do this. What's more, you'll find it easier to resist food cravings because you will be able to stay present with your feelings and to make different choices.

THE WILLINGNESS TO FEEL

Once you are able to bring your body back to the safety of the relaxation state, you will be able to experience a whole range of feelings. You will find that you are less numb in general. I used to think that antidepressants eliminated depression until a psychiatrist explained to me that antidepressants take away our capacity to feel emotions, the good and the bad. This is what food can do as well. As Ariel White told me, true pleasure is sensitizing, while counterfeit pleasure is desensitizing. When we numb ourselves with food, it is a counterfeit pleasure that works like insulation, distancing us from both our painful and our pleasurable feelings. The Pleasurable Weight Loss approach is about removing the insulation so that we feel more sensations across the board. If you've felt stuck in your weight and habits with food, it's time to realize that you've been reacting to the conditioned limits of your nervous system, which dictate your pleasure threshold.

When you become more open to feeling in general, you'll also find that you are more aware of pain. We can't selectively choose to feel only more of the good feelings, but this doesn't mean that we will have more pain than before or that we are stuck with it. On the contrary, fully feeling your pain is the fastest way to move it out of your body and mind. Hand in hand with our capacity to experience pleasure in a grounded and open way is our capacity to experience pain with the same presence and open-heartedness. This is what's known as resilience. If you can bear your pain, or face any of the feelings you are trying to avoid, the knee-jerk reaction to avoid such emotions by eating will be dissolved. When you are present to your wounds, the regenerative principle of life is triggered, and you begin to heal.

When I first learned to self-regulate my nervous system through yoga, I also found myself more able to be present with my emotions. As this happened, I discovered layers of hidden trauma I had shoved under the proverbial rug of my psyche. In the past, these feelings had been too intense to deal with on my own, and I was ashamed to reveal my pain to anyone. Instead, I numbed myself to my feelings until years later, when through yoga I finally had both the tools and the community support that enabled me to feel my pain, face my demons, and heal my wounds.

No matter what you have been through, you can meet your painful feelings head-on. At first, it can feel like the pain is endless. You may be afraid that if you allow yourself to surrender to your feelings, you will cry forever, but at a certain point, your tears will dry up. Facing our painful feelings provides an incredible opportunity to grow.

In addition to the widely known post-traumatic stress disorder (PTSD), there is another response to trauma known as post-traumatic growth. This is the positive growth trauma that survivors—such as those who have experienced military combat, a natural disaster, abuse, sexual assault, or chronic illness—can experience. Instead of emerging from trauma disassociated from their bodies and their lives, they are more finely attuned to feeling. They report greater openness, heightened spirituality, greater compassion, and enhanced personal strength and self-confidence. They also report heightened intimacy and a greater appreciation for their relationships.

Your struggle with food and your body image is a trauma. Layers of pain will reveal themselves in the process of moving more profoundly into pleasure. As you confront each layer, you have the choice to contract into a PTSD response or to use tools for self-regulation and grounding to expand into post-traumatic growth instead.

What it takes to learn to melt pain quickly and return to a state of relaxation is willingness. Javier Regueiro describes the difference between willpower (the all-too-familiar vehicle of the masculine punishing strategies) and willingness (a secret ingredient in the feminine pleasurable approach): "Willingness implies both the active part of doing whatever is needed, as in willpower, as well as a surrendering and embracing of whatever is really laying in front of us that can probably use our attention." In other words, instead of attempting to barrel through the pain your body has been holding, which has prevented you from losing weight, shift to a willingness that includes facing whatever is needed along the way, even if it's challenging.

Amy Dawn Verebay says, "Embracing your pain is important because when it comes up, we think it's bottomless. We think it's going to kill us and that it has an enormous power beyond our knowing that could destroy us. But when you know that anger, for example, is a part of life, and so is fear, and they ebb and flow, and they're just part of this pulsation that is the totality of life, meant to be experienced and felt, then it puts you in a place of peace."

When you fill your life with pleasure, it can fortify you with the courage to sit with pain and to feel it through all the way to the end. Feeling more is a process of getting to know yourself, during which you will discover the nooks and crannies of your being, physically and emotionally. "I am willing," is the mantra Javier recommends we repeat whenever we are faced with sensations that threaten to overcome our sense of safety. This mantra is useful for moments when the intense sensation of a situation threatens to trigger you into fear and the stress response.

Once you are able to face your painful emotions, you are also ready to actively nudge the edges of your pleasure threshold, so that you can experience greater heights of pleasure. When you are faced with intense sensations, take deep breaths all the way down to your belly, with a longer exhalation than inhalation, which relaxes your nervous system. By doing so, you will gradually unwind old stressful patterns and begin to lift your pleasure threshold. Equipped to feel more fully and deeply, you can now dissolve the old patterns without drowning yourself in food.

Nestled between the black-and-white polarities of safe and unsafe lies a gray zone, where the sensations dance on the edge between comfort and discomfort. When an experience feels edgy, it can require your complete awareness to prevent setting off trip-wires of the stress response or diffusing the experience with a distraction. Feeling this edge is an indicator that you are bumping up against your limits.

One of the secrets of pleasurable weight loss is knowing how to respond in these moments when you meet an edge. For example, overeating might feel comfortable and safe for you: even if it's not good for you, it's a familiar sensation. Similarly, if you are used to eating all of your meals in front of the television, sitting down to a meal at a table free of distractions might feel uncomfortable and unsafe. Even though it's good for you, it's an unfamiliar sensation. These would be your current pleasure thresholds. Your task is to expand the thresholds so that you can increase the range of pleasurable sensations available to you. To lift your pleasure threshold, you need to bring your conscious awareness to the sensations of pleasure as they occur and tolerate them. When you do this, the reptilian brain will recalibrate what it knows as safe. Your comfort with the new sensation will grow.

Women's sexuality expert Saida Désilets, PhD, describes the moment of consciously arriving at your pleasure threshold: "Give yourself a moment to notice, 'Ah, I'm sitting on an edge. This is my pleasure threshold, I've reached it.' Then, just sit there and give yourself space. You don't have to make a decision. It's really a beautiful experience where you are not pushing yourself in either direction; you are just allowing yourself to be there. Sometimes that's enough to make you ready to expand beyond an edge. Sometimes you will think, 'I'm not quite ready for that yet.' Whatever we choose, it's vital we trust our instinctual wisdom."

When you come into contact with an edgy sensation, notice what the sensation actually feels like, without ascribing judgment or meaning. By doing so, you can decouple the sensation from its meaning and give it a new name or label that simply describes what is happening on the physical level. The secret to mastering this ability to dance on the edge between the known and the unknown is being willing to meet sensation on its own terms, without the interference of the mind. For example, if you are feeling anxious, stop for a moment and see if you can describe to yourself what the anxiety really feels like. It might feel like heat in the belly, tightness in the chest, pressure above the eyebrows, or all three at once. Get curious about the unique texture and form of the sensation. This helps you to dismantle the mental constructs of your interpretation of the sensation, so you can be fully aware of the entirety of the feeling and how it may change. You will find that sensations never stay the same for long; they are continuously morphing into something different.

The ability to separate sensations from the meanings you usually give these sensations (such as "this sensation means I need a cookie") is liberating. When you can dissolve your previous interpretation of a sensation that led you to overeat, you can respond differently the next time it occurs. By being present with the sensation, you won't abandon your connection with your female animal and run to the cookie jar; instead, you'll know that what you are feeling is only a sensation that will quickly pass.

As another example, if you're experiencing anxiety, instead of putting your attention on the fact that you are experiencing anxiety, rest your attention on the changing sensations in your body, each defined by its own visceral quality. When you can reduce your anxiety to these sensations, you will no longer find yourself in the grip of the story that had been justifying them, and the anxiety will lose its power over you. It will become just another feeling.

Embodiment expert Michaela Boehm teaches that when we meet our edge, developing our capacity for positive self-talk is critical: "Anytime you feel unsafe or on the edge of your pleasure threshold, but there is no actual danger, you need to be able to say to yourself, 'It's okay. I'm a grown woman now. This is good. Nothing dangerous is happening right now. I can do it. I'm okay.' "

When you walk yourself lovingly and supportively along the edge of your pleasure threshold, over time the boundary moves, and the range of what feels safe to you expands. When you've made it through to the other side, just as you would commend a child, you need to give yourself the same positive reinforcement: "See, that was fine. You did it. That was no problem."

Learning to expand your tolerance for pleasure is an essential secret of pleasurable weight loss. The broader the range of sensations you are able to tolerate, the more expansive highs of pleasure you will experience. What's more, you'll be able to handle the intensities of life without defaulting to the stress response. By expanding your comfort zone, you'll stay more grounded, be better able to cope, and be more relaxed more of the time, even in the face of difficult or negative experiences. You'll also become more confident that you can manage uncomfortable feelings without overeating.

By lifting your pleasure threshold, you will be able to sustain a wider range of sensations. For example, a woman who finds it uncomfortable to be touched can learn how to relax into a full body massage, or a woman who has never had an orgasm can expand to have multiple orgasms. The pleasure you get from any realm in life can exponentially increase. Executive advisor and coach Jennifer Russell likes to say, "Range is God," implying that more than any one specific quality, what is truly divine is the ability to experience the whole spectrum of sensations. My wish for you is that you be able to fully feel and embody the full spectrum of womanhood.

PLEASURE PRACTICE
Expand Your Range

Something as simple as your daily shower can be an oppor-tunity to practice range. Instead of setting the water only at the comfortable temperature you know and love, exper-iment with the temperature. Go to the edge of your heat tolerance and then to your cold tolerance. Go back and forth a few times. On a physiological level, this will cause your capillaries to expand and contract, which boosts your cir-culation and detoxifies your lymph nodes. On an emotional level, it will show you that you can reach your tolerance for intensity without tipping into stress mode. The next time you are faced with a situation where there's more at stake than the comfortable temperature of your shower, you will have more confidence in your ability to weather the sensa-tions that come your way.

THE FEMININE TRAIT OF BEHAVIORAL FLEXIBILITY

Another way to describe range is "behavioral flexibility." While the punishing strategies for weight loss urge you to take more control over the situation, the pleasurable strategy advocates flex-ibility in your behavior. This approach stems from a feminine understanding of control, which is that the most flexible aspect of a system controls the system.

Behavioral flexibility relates directly to accountability and the process of authoring your life. When you are confident in your range of behaviors, you have boundless options with which to respond to any situation. For example, if a situation usually triggers you to overeat, behavioral flexibility will allow you to make a different choice. With regard to your body image, behavioral flexibility means that you can interrupt a stream of critical judgments about your body and redirect your mind to thoughts that are compassionate and kind. And in the realms of sensuality and sexuality, imagine how much more fun and excitement behavioral flexibility can bring to your relationships!

Behavioral flexibility depends on your ability to be present, to be aware of sensations without defaulting into the fight-or-flight mode. By learning to hold more sensation in your body, when you are faced with a situation in which you may have been vulnerable to overeating in the past, you'll now possess the ability to stay grounded, with a deeper intention for your female animal, and to respond to the sensation with a different behavior that serves you better. When you have a greater tolerance for sensation, you can increase your capacity to stay present with hunger. Whereas before, the slightest twinge of hunger might have sent you searching for an easy snack, a greater tolerance for sensation will allow you to stay grounded and to sit with hunger without reacting compulsively to the sensation. Then, when you feel cravings for foods you know don't serve your animal, you can tap into behavioral options and choose to do something else, like getting up and walking around, having a dance break, or drinking a glass of water. And when you do choose to eat, you can make a healthier choice.

PLEASURE PRACTICE
Facing Your Cravings

When we are open to be with both our physical sensations and our feelings, we can face our cravings and separate the sensations from the thoughts we've assigned to them. Embodiment teacher Amber Hartnell taught me this next practice. When you are facing a craving to eat junk food or to binge, the first move is to stop and catch yourself midstream in the throes of your habituated pattern. Instead of thinking, "Oh my God! This craving is so intense I can't handle ignoring it," get curious about it and begin to unpack the sensation. Does it feel prickly? Sharp? Is it tingling? Throbbing? Bring your attention to the sensation and breathe it open. Breathe love, appreciation, and softness into it.

Instead of allowing the mental chatter of your mind's judgments to dictate a story about what is happening, stay with your awareness of the sensations themselves, which will eventually bring you to a neutral space. Soften into your belly, and then from the inside begin to melt the body open so that a state of relaxed alertness meets the discomfort. Even in a moment when you want to run from the sensation, with enough presence, the intensity can be dissolved.

Then, check a little more deeply and ask your animal, "Do I really need to eat this?" This is when you can make a different choice. You can interrupt the craving and redirect it in any direction you desire. You can redirect it by asking, "What would actually be nourishing for me right now? What would be inspiring?" In effect, you are discovering what will bring her the greatest pleasure. You may find that there's something more nourishing available once you are willing to stay with the feeling. Instead of turning away from discomfort, let the sensation propel you in another direction, where the craving can be fulfilled in healthy ways.

THE FEMININE GIFT OF HUMOR

Losing weight is about lightening up, which includes lightening up emotionally. One of the most effective ways to lighten your mood is the pleasurable weight loss secret of humor. When you realize that you have been taking yourself and life far too seriously, you free yourself to get in touch with your inner clown and to find the divine comedy of the moment. I spent decades taking myself way too seriously. Whether it was obsessing over my body image or working crazy hours, I was stressed out, dried up, and lonely. I found that being too serious boxed me in when my soul really wanted to break out and play.

There's magic in learning to laugh at ourselves. Anytime we find ourselves in the grip of the stress response, we can reach for humor to lighten things up.

Watch a funny movie, go to a comedy show, or spend time with friends who make you laugh. Find ways to be silly and ridiculous.

SENSUALITY IS YOUR BIRTHRIGHT

Another feminine value is sensuality, opening up to experience the world through the riches of the senses—taste, touch, smell, sound, and sight. The senses are the language of the feminine, and ultimately the gateway to pleasure. Our senses must be experienced in order to fully embody pleasure. If we are numb to them, we're missing a critical opportunity to feel fully alive. Every sense offers a unique avenue for pleasure.

Many people think of pleasures in the extreme, like a big piece of chocolate cake or a mind-blowing orgasm. But sensuality teaches us that pleasures can be found in the small and subtle things, if we only take the time to allow our senses to be tickled. Frequently, women fear that letting themselves live through their senses will lead them straight to the Boston cream pies or the all-you-can-eat buffet, but those who actually do that quickly discover that overeating isn't the sensually gratifying experience they expected it to be. Sensual experiences encompass so much more than what we put into our mouths.

There are endless ways that you can connect with your sensuality. Take your time, be curious, and enjoy discovering them. Sensuality is linked to slowly discovering the small things in life through the senses. These can include wearing silk lingerie, anointing yourself with a favorite perfume, cooking a meal that fills the kitchen with the aromas of spices and herbs, dancing, and taking a leisurely stroll outdoors.

Although it is common for women to believe they will feel more sensual once they lose weight, my years of coaching experience have shown that the opposite is true: it's when women become more attentive to their sensuality first that it acts as a powerful catalyst for slimming down. When you are connected to your sensuality, you have a direct connection to your body, your intuition, and your authentic desires.

My client April, a human resources director at a large corporation, told me that her work life was anything but sensual. She worked such long hours that by the time she got home, all she could think about was eating ice cream because she felt so sensually deprived. Looking for ways to bring sensuality to her day, we included a focus on increasing the pleasure of every meal. I told April that she needed to take a lunch break away from her desk, a real lunch break that allowed her to drop into her senses while she was feeding her animal. She followed my advice and implemented Pleasurable Eating Practices at lunch. The next time she saw me, April reported feeling more grounded and less affected by nightly cravings. Prioritizing sensuality helped her lose weight, whereas trying to discipline herself to eat less never did.

THE PLEASURE OF TOUCH

One of the best ways to expand your tolerance for sensation and get back in touch with sensuality at the same time is through massage. If you are uncomfortable with being touched, it is time to change that by diving into the beautiful art of giving and receiving a massage. The first time I encountered the healing powers of massage, it changed my life. Apart from sleeping, it was the first time my body had been so fully relaxed—to the point of euphoria. Still feeling the energizing effects of the experience the next day, I made a decision that massage would be a regular part of my life. In the spirit of what goes around comes around, it seemed obvious to me that the most reliable way to be on the receiving end of a massage would be to learn how to give one. I learned how to tap into my intuitive ability to feel into someone's muscles and offer her relief and relaxation. Since then, in addition to receiving professional massages, I've enjoyed many informal massage exchanges with friends, which have brought great pleasure into my life.

We all know that giving a massage takes skill, but it's a little-known fact that receiving a massage also takes skill—skill that supports pleasurable weight loss. Anyone can lie down on a massage table and passively be touched; however, this is not the same as skillfully receiving the maximum pleasure and benefits of a massage. Good receivers allow touch to melt them like butter; they engage in full relaxation. Bad receivers don't fully let go; subtly or not so subtly, they resist being touched. Skillful receiving requires putting yourself in a mind-set of trust so that you can surrender your body to the touch of another. In a culture where mistrust of the body is pervasive, learning to receive a massage is one way to regain that trust.

When you receive a massage, you are the only one who knows if it feels good—whether the touch is too hard, too soft, too fast, or too slow. Only you can provide feedback, verbally or nonverbally, to the massage therapist. As you develop your ability to tell someone what you like and what you don't like when you're being touched—not based on a concept of what you think feels good but on what actually opens you to pleasure—you're on the path to mastering that skill elsewhere in your life. When you know what feels really good to your body and you trust yourself enough to let others know, you'll feel more confident deciding what to eat, how to move, and then how to live to support losing weight pleasurably and feeling at peace with food.

During a massage, your body is flooded with the same pleasure chemistry that heightens calorie-burning efficiency. The side effects of a good massage include elevating your mood, enhancing your immune system, and stimulating your libido. When your mood is high, your body feels strong, and you feel your sexual potency flowing in your veins; you're in a state where you're less likely to fulfill your pleasure needs at the fridge.

The more you explore giving and receiving massage, the more sensual and relaxing your experience will be. Learning the body mechanics of giving a massage will teach you how not to strain your hands, neck, and back, as well as how to feel rejuvenated by a massage even when you are the giver. When giving in this way becomes pleasurable, you will develop a new area of self-esteem. You will feel confident in your skill as a pleasure giver, which goes hand in hand with knowing you are worthy of receiving pleasure. While women generally don't need to be reminded to give, developing a high regard for yourself as someone who is talented at giving as well as receiving pleasure improves how you feel about yourself. By taking pleasure in giving and receiving massage, you'll be more connected with your body, more connected with other people, and more confident in your ability to design and live a life of pleasure.

PLEASURE PRACTICE
Giving and Receiving Touch

We all naturally crave touch, yet in the isolating digital age, many of us are starved of this pleasure. Touch is the first pleasure every mother shares with her child, and it continues to have the power to immediately bring us into the present. Good touch is, of course, relaxing, and it brings our awareness out of our heads and into our bodies.

Be proactive about making touch a part of your life. Treat yourself to a professional massage or ask a loved one to massage you. During a massage, practice letting go of the mental thought loops that may be circling in your mind and bring your attention back to your body. Deepening your breath is a great way to start to feel more and think less. Allow your awareness to stay with the sensation of the touch on your body, which will give your thinking mind a chance to rest and reboot. Instead of chatting during the massage, see if you can drop into a nonverbal space. While words of appreciation to the giver are lovely, rather than becoming too verbal, which is distracting, express your pleasure and gratitude through moans, groans, and sighs of delight.

I also encourage you to be generous with your touch and to be physically affectionate with your friends and loved ones. Be the initiator of exchanging foot or shoulder rubs—maybe even exchanging a full-body massage. Notice how much pleasure you can take from giving. And remember not to abandon your own animal when your attention is on giving pleasure to someone else.

PLEASURE BITE

A light touch can be intensely pleasurable. A wonderful tool for experiencing the power of delicate touch is an ostrich feather. Buy one to keep next to your bed, and use it to slowly caress your skin.

5 PLEASURABLE EATING PRACTICE 5
Seek Pleasure in Every Bite

You are now ready to eat. You'll find that when you eat with pleasure, incredible things happen. You smile, relax, and appreciate the beauty of who you are. All your senses come alive, and you are more present to the world. You signal your metabolism to ramp up your calorie-burning efficiency because you're not in a stress state.

When you eat with sensuality, you heighten the pleasure of the meal by slowing down and deliberately savoring the experience through your senses. Continue to check in with your animal, bite by bite, to make sure that you are still receiving pleasure from the eating experience. When you eat with presence, you will hear her voice loud and clear. If you don't pay attention to the pleasure of every bite, you miss out on the sensation of her letting you know when you've had enough to eat.

The aim is to extract as much pleasure from the food and the eating experience as you can to heighten your metabolism. Remember, your animal doesn't speak in the language of calories or numbers. But she can sense what the right amount of food for you is. To maximize the pleasure, pay attention to the taste, smell, and texture of the food, and feel the way your body reacts to it. Become acutely aware of the sensuality of the food entering your mouth. This will activate your body's pleasure chemistry and its natural appetite.

RECLAIMING YOUR FEMININE BEAUTY

Just as you deserve pleasure every day, you deserve to feel and look beautiful, starting right now. It may have been deeply impressed upon you that beauty is only what models portray and that you will never measure up, no matter how hard you try. Beauty may feel like something other women have. In comparison, you may feel heavier, flabbier, and maybe more wrinkled. The list goes on—but that's only because you've been judging your beauty by the media's definition, which is of course an unattainable standard aimed to keep you buying products that promise to make you look better while the companies secure their profits.

Although the women we see in the media may be beautiful, they do not represent the sole definition of beauty. We know this because diverse cultures define beauty differently. Scan the continents and you'll find a new definition of beauty wherever you go. Imagine seeing your own image for the first time through eyes influenced by a global perspective. You might find that you admire your nose; appreciate your hair; find the charm in your smile; or love your breasts, hips, and thighs. As unhappy as you may be about your weight, each of us has a distinct beauty and style.

Another secret to pleasurable weight loss is the feeling of being beautiful, which is available to every woman. You just need to claim it. As Mama Gena says, "Ownership is the key to beauty. You gotta dig on down and own yours to have yours. Every Sister Goddess—no matter how beautiful she is—has to know and accept herself if she is to get hold of her own special brand of beauty, if she is to truly own it. Loving ourselves releases our life force and expands our beauty. Our innate beauty is nothing without enthusiasm backing it up."

I endorse an earth-based definition of beauty, which is broader, more natural, and more feminine. Whereas a masculine approach to beauty focuses on the details, the feminine approach embraces the big picture of our beauty. The trick is to keep a feminine holistic view of your beauty in mind and not to go down the rabbit hole of masculine analysis—which makes you vulnerable to lasering in on your perceived flaws, such as cellulite or stretch marks. For example, even though I've been able to maintain my weight loss for over ten years, from time to time, I notice critical thoughts about my body creep into my head. When this happens, I consciously silence those voices by returning my attention to the ways my body feels good. At the end of the day, defining beauty and feeling good about ourselves is an inside job.

You may also feel conflicted by beauty: a part of you may yearn for it, while another considers it a shallow pursuit. But don't be. All beauty in life is a reflection of nature's perfection. Just as a flower is naturally beautiful, so are you. Your beauty is a gift to be embraced without the slightest hint of shame. It is to be relished and enjoyed. When I am complimented for my beauty, I bow inwardly to Mother Nature and allow myself to be revitalized in my service to humanity.

PLEASURE PRACTICE
Claiming Your Beauty

If you've ever thought, "Who am I to be beautiful?" listen up. The answer is "Who am I not to be beautiful?" The first step to knowing that in your bones is to evolve your conception of beauty beyond the masculine, media-defined standard. Mama Gena teaches us that loving all the features we have—the perfect, the quirky, and the imperfect—is the secret to feeling beautiful. To choose to feel beautiful, no matter what, takes great tenacity. She writes, "We all have access to the glow of gorgeousness. The question becomes, how interested are we in being beautiful? Are we interested enough to accept ourselves completely in order to be a knockout?" Now is the time to claim your beauty. Stand in front of a mirror and give yourself a compliment, and take pleasure in it! Internalizing this kind appreciation creates a radiance that is universally beautiful.

MAKING YOUR WHOLE LIFE BEAUTIFUL

Beauty is a complete philosophy of living. Annie Lalla teaches that the philosophy of beauty requires taking responsibility for creating your own aesthetic criteria for life, to include people, places, and things you appreciate and admire, as well as the world of ideas, thoughts, and feelings. Too many women fail to be conscious about their aesthetics. They are too busy taking care of others or seeking approval to realize the importance of investing time in nourishing themselves. Because they do not bring enough attention to curating their reality, they end up leading lives high in stress and low in beauty.

However, once you commit to actively engage your beauty filters, everything changes. Home in on what would make your life more beautiful—don't let this be vague and undefined. For example, when your beauty filter has been reset to sort for fresh and nourishing ingredients, junk food may no longer make it past your lips. When it has been reset to find inspiring, pleasure-positive friends, the company of people who drain your energy may cease to be acceptable. When you are surrounded by beauty and pleasure, you'll be able to see and feel the beauty within yourself so profoundly that you will no longer be able to deny that you, too, are gorgeous!

Before you start worrying about a right or a wrong way to do this, remember that no aesthetic is better than any other. You might be attracted to clothes made from all natural fibers or stretchy synthetic spandex. In your bedroom, you might love double-lined curtains that keep the sun out because you like to sleep late or breezy white curtains that let in the first light of day. What matters is that you own your aesthetic. What a relief it is to be freed from fulfilling anyone else's definition of beauty because you are securely grounded in your own, across every dimension of your life.

To feel congruent owning your beauty on the outside, you must first feel that you are a beautiful person on the inside. One of the reasons you may want to lose weight is to build your self-esteem, but self-esteem can't be found in a number on the scale. It's when you recognize your inner beauty and the beauty of the existence you are authoring that your self-esteem skyrockets and boosts how good you feel about your body—all of which ultimately stimulates weight loss. One technique to cultivate your esteem, which I learned from Annie Lalla, is to focus on what you admire about yourself. This is a radical act that invites you to investigate, even if you are a hundred pounds overweight, what is beautiful about you. It could be the way you walk, your smile, your hair, or your curves. It could be that you write well, have an eye for design, or easily make new friends. Let this habit of noticing what you admire about yourself and approving of your beauty be yet another aspect that you love about yourself.

You don't have to be perfect in any of these areas to be admirable. Setting perfection as your standard is severely limiting because anything that falls short of perfection will be another source of disappointment and stress. This is why some people never try anything new; they're afraid that they won't be able to attain perfection, so why go there? When it comes to weight loss, too, many women don't try because they believe that they'll never have "the perfect body" anyway. What they don't realize is that they are putting the idea of a perfect body on an altar, as if this standard possessed a divine quality superior to where they are now or could ever be. Worshipping perfection is a misdirected search for the divine, and looking for the divine in a future goal will cause you to miss out on experiencing the divine here and now. But when you consciously let go of the mental construct of perfectionism, you can relax into enjoying your body and your life now and throughout your journey. Because there is no such thing as perfection, when you can embrace your "imperfection" as an aspect of your unique beauty, you'll fall in love with yourself right now.

PLEASURE PRACTICE
Create Your Own Beauty Standards

This exercise prompts you to create your own beauty aesthetic. List the criteria that define a beautiful existence for you in the realms of body, mind, heart, character, actions, and environments. What defines the beauty you would be attracted to and inspired to live? For every choice you make in your day and in your life, choose according to your aesthetics.

PLEASURE BITE

Turn your bedroom into a beautiful and sensual boudoir, a sanctuary that honors your feminine energy. Choose colors, fabrics, lighting, aromas, music, etc., that enhance your daily experience of pleasure and relaxation.

THE POWER OF CREATIVITY

When you embrace your feminine nature, you realize that you are creative to the bone and can bring those powers to any area of your life. Creativity is crucial for pleasurable weight loss for multiple reasons. Without a creative outlet for the expression of your feelings and emotions, they will be bottled up, and then it's only a matter of time until they become a trigger for overeating. When you express yourself creatively, you boost your self-esteem. By making a regular practice of engaging your creativity in any context, when you are faced with difficult situations that once may have led you to overeat to drown your sorrows, you'll instead have access to creative solutions for whatever challenges you face. When you are in the present moment and connected with your animal, your creativity awakens. Being willing to experience any sensation, emotion, or experience stimulates your creative potential.

PLEASURE PRACTICE
Getting Your Creative Juices Going

Think of creativity as another facet of your body's natural appetite, which has been pushed underground. Make creative expression a non-negotiable priority in your week. What form of creativity do you hunger for, or at least have curiosity about? What were your creative outlets as a child? Can you revive any of them? Write a list of all the creative outlets that interest you.

In the family of thieves, the child who will not steal
has a guilty conscience.

BERT HELLINGER

6 Creating the Ideal Ecology for Pleasurable Weight Loss

ALL FORMS OF LIFE are supported by their unique ecosystem, or ecology. Yours includes both your external environment and your inner world. Your ecology includes your family, where you buy your food, and what's in your refrigerator and pantry. It's where and how you eat, as well as the people you socialize with. It's what goes on in your head and heart—what you believe, what you think, and what you value. All of the factors that makeup your outer and inner worlds influence your present circumstances, your status quo. In this chapter, I'm going to teach you another essential secret to pleasurable weight loss: unless you attend to your ecology, any changes you make regarding food and your weight will be the equivalent of stretching a rubber band: you will take on a new shape but soon snap back to where you began.

A masculine approach to weight loss sets your eye on a goal and plots the fastest way to get there, but the feminine, pleasurable approach is more akin to growing a flower in a garden. You start by creating the right ecology, which begins with a vision of the flower you wish to see bloom. Even before you plant the seed, you prepare and fertilize the soil. Once you plant the seed, you water the earth, wait for sunshine, and keep faith that the seed will sprout. You nurture the seedling with appreciation and joy as it grows, and lo and behold, without rushing or cajoling, the flower blossoms in its own time. We are going to work together along similar lines to create the right ecology for you to experience pleasurable weight loss.

Punishing diets fail because they focus only on the outcome of weight loss and not on the ecology. But just as you would support a flower's growth by paying attention to the conditions of the garden, you have to evolve the world you live in and your sense of self before you can lose weight. This ecological approach requires examining every aspect of your life, as you weed out the obstacles that cause stress and prevent you from losing weight. Some of the beliefs within your current ecology are well intentioned but misguided, and holding on to them will keep you feeling heavy and struggling with food forever. Redesigning your ecology to support your weight loss is about letting go of the old— such as judgments, resentments, anger, hurt, and other painful emotions that stand in the way of pleasure—as well as bringing in the new.

If you're struggling with food and weight, then your ecology clearly is not supporting you. Instead of focusing on food as the problem, the feminine approach takes a wide view to look at the big picture of what is really going on. This approach guides you to create a new ecology that will serve you better.

PLEASURE PRACTICE
Optimizing Your External Ecology

If you could design your external environment to meet your animal's ideal conditions, what would it look and feel like? You can make both your home and work ecologies more relaxing and supportive of your body. Among the elements you tend to, consider the temperature of your home and office, the way the air circulates, the aroma in the air, the colors of the space, the quality of the lighting, the level of clutter, and the decorative touches that make you feel your best.

BECOMING A NATURALLY SLENDER WOMAN

You may have assumed that you will never be one of those women who can maintain a slim figure. Or you may think that it is in your grasp but that it will take great willpower and a lot of work. But this is not the case at all. Given the right ecology, you can become what weight loss expert Renée Stephens, PhD, author of *Ful-filled,* so elegantly describes as a naturally slender person.

It is easy to buy into the myth that being slim is available to some women but not others. The truth is, we all come into the world with the knowledge of what to eat when we're hungry and how to stop when we're satisfied. But along the way we start disconnecting from our animal and start eating for reasons other than hunger. Yet no matter how out of touch you may have gotten from your instinctive wisdom, it's hardwired and can't be lost. It's completely possible to reconnect with the voice of your female animal so that you can easily become naturally slender, even if you currently struggle with compulsive eating.

Being a naturally slender woman takes no willpower, no effort, no control, and requires no deprivation when you experience a fundamental ease that comes from being in tune with your female animal. You listen and respond to your body's messages and signals, not just for hunger and satiety but also for all other levels of self-care and nourishment. Effortlessly maintaining a weight that feels fabulous is the goal of pleasurable weight loss. The last thing I want is for your weight to be another thing on your to-do list. I want you to completely transcend the paradigm of being on or off a diet and to be living your life simply, in an abundance of healthy pleasure and in a naturally slender body that is a side effect of a sustainable ecology that supports you.

PLEASURE PRACTICE
What Are You Hoping Losing Weight Will Do for You?

The next step in creating a new ecology is to discern your real intention for losing weight. What will losing weight do for you? The answers may well include feeling good, looking good, getting out into the world, being more colorful, enjoying clothes, feeling more powerful or active, enjoying your body, and loving yourself. Write down your answers.

Now that you have this list, you can start to put your attention toward achieving these desires by making them part of your ecology. How can you have the experience you are looking for even before you lose the weight? It might begin with a mind-set shift, or it might involve a change in lifestyle.

RAT PARK

The lab results seemed to be unequivocal: if you give rats addicted to morphine the opportunity to drink water or water laced with morphine, they will keep dosing themselves with morphine until they die. The takeaway lesson clearly showed the addictive nature of morphine. That was until psychologist and researcher Bruce Alexander ruffled feathers by challenging the whole paradigm of the experiment. He asked a valid question: "Who wouldn't medicate themselves with morphine if confined to the distressing ecology of a lab cage?"

To test his hypothesis, Alexander built Rat Park, a rat's paradise in comparison to the typical research cage. Rat Park was two hundred times larger, included rats of both sexes, had an abundance of food, toys to play with, nooks and crannies to rest in, and ample space for mating—as well as water and water laced with morphine. Based on the previous results, we would expect the addicted rats to continue to self-administer morphine until they died. However, that wasn't what happened. For the most part, the rats in Rat Park chose the plain water and weaned themselves off the morphine, or they used the morphine water sparingly. Alexander showed that ecology matters.

Applying the same principle to our own lives, the moral of the story is that we can vilify carbs or fat for being tempting and addictive or vilify ourselves for being unable to refuse the urge, but neither is the culprit. Instead, we need to view our intense cravings and weight struggle as a sign that our current ecology is distressing so we are medicating to compensate. The remedy is to address our ecology, making it truly pleasurable so that an excess of food will no longer be needed.

PLEASURE BITE

Your animal enjoys being hydrated. You can make this a sensual experience by filling a beautiful jug with water and adding some citrus slices. Have a bowl of fresh fruit on your counter so your animal always has a healthy snack on hand. Simple changes like these will improve your ecology and support pleasurable weight loss.

UNLEASHING YOUR OLD ECOLOGY:
THE POWER OF YOUR POSITIVE INTENTIONS

Behind every one of our behaviors, even overeating and gaining weight, is an unconscious positive intention. It is the hidden motivation that drives us toward an experience. Though at first glance it seems overeating is a self-destructive habit, when we look more deeply, there is always something we gain by being overweight—something we would potentially lose if we lost the weight and came to peace with food. These hidden benefits are also known as secondary gains. To uncover your motivations, examine what you are currently receiving from your extra weight and eating habits, so that you can get those same needs fulfilled in healthier ways.

You are not overeating because you are flawed, broken, or weak. You are doing it because you want to create a good feeling for yourself. You want to move toward pleasure and away from pain. This pain might be something as primary as the discomfort of being with yourself. It could be any number of struggles in your life, even shame about overeating. It's not your fault you've been turning to food. In a culture that frowns upon a woman's sensuality and sexuality, that has us disconnected from nature, isolated from our sisters, where else were you going to turn for pleasure? Overeating was a fairly reasonable strategy for bringing yourself pleasure. Some people make riskier choices, like heroin or gambling, to feel good. Wanting to feel good is a beautiful urge, and as we've seen, seeking pleasure is not the problem. It's how you've been going about eating that makes it a suboptimal strategy, driven by a pure positive intention.

Maybe you decided that gaining weight was the best way to deflect undesired attention. If you have been emotionally, physically, or sexually hurt or abused, extra weight is an obvious form of protection because weight can literally protect us from physical harm. Extra weight is also the unconscious mind's way of keeping you safe, even from your own uncomfortable feelings, such as anger, rage, hurt, or betrayal. It can protect you sexually by keeping men away, and it can protect you emotionally by keeping others distant. Extra weight can numb uncomfortable feelings and past hurts, and it can distract us from important issues in our relationships or careers that need our attention.

Again, there's nothing bad or wrong about being where you are now because you made the best choices available to you at the time. There's no need to be ashamed because there were underlying positive intentions. You can even be proud of yourself. At the root, you've been trying to stay safe, and that's admirable and wise. Although you now feel that being overweight is a problem and no longer aligned with what you want, in the past it was a brilliant solution.

It has been my observation that we always get what we want in life, if attaining it will bring more benefits than disadvantages. I call this theory The Scales of Getting What You Want. To understand this idea, imagine you have old-fashioned weighing scales, the kind that symbolize justice. On one side, you weigh all the benefits you'd get from attaining what you want; on the other side, all the drawbacks. If you have more on the side of benefits, you get what you want, and if you have more on the side of disadvantages, you don't.

When I share with my clients and workshop participants the idea that they would have already lost weight and resolved their food struggle if it brought them more benefits than drawbacks, they typically regard me with a puzzled look. "What on earth could be the drawbacks of losing weight?" they inevitably ask. "I see only benefits."

"Let's start with the benefits then," I reply. "What good do you hope to gain from losing weight?" I ask them.

In the blink of an eye out comes a long list: I'd have more energy, I'd feel healthier, I'd feel more beautiful, I'd be happier, I'd have more sex, I'd have more peace of mind, I could fit into anything and buying clothes would be easier and more fun, I'd be more attractive to my partner, or (for the single ladies) I'd attract my dream mate. These answers get written on the right side of the scales, which is illustrated below.

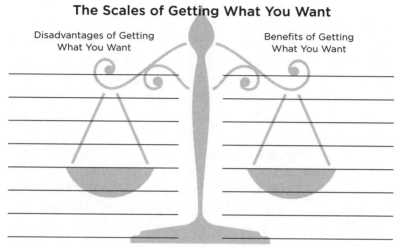

The Scales of Getting What You Want

Disadvantages of Getting
What You Want

Benefits of Getting
What You Want

figure 5

Next, I ask a more probing question: "So let's say you've lost the weight you desire. What might you lose that you value?" At first, they look at me with blank stares. "Are you nuts? I wouldn't lose anything I value!" Undeterred, I invite them to dig deeper to investigate the positive intentions beneath their current weight and relationship with food. "What might be the cost you secretly fear that will be part of getting what you want?"

One woman will eventually break the silence with something like, "Well, if I lost weight, I'd lose my favorite way of comforting myself." All it takes is one, and then the whole room erupts with more insights: "I'd lose the freedom to eat whatever I want."

"I'd need to cook more and I don't like cooking." "Maintaining my figure would be hard work." "If I lost weight and gained it back, I'd be mortified." "I'd lose my default excuse for the things I'm scared to do." "If I felt really good about myself, I might not be willing to put up with my husband's negativity, and I might lose my marriage." "It would change my relationship with other people." "I'd feel pressure to keep it off." "It would be expensive." "I'd get lots of attention." "I'd lose my weapon of revenge." "My mother/sister/friends would be jealous." "My husband would be threatened." "I'd lose my safety."

These answers go on the left side of the scales. Then, we compare the two sides. Once these answers have been uncovered, my clients become aware of the many ways that their weight has been benefitting them. Now they are ready to begin the process of forgiving themselves, releasing shame, and starting a new, more direct, and mature relationship with food and weight.

I have never met a woman who, when she was honest with herself, was not able to see that although she wants to lose weight, on a subconscious level there are more reasons she doesn't want to lose weight, which were holding her back. Understanding this concept of positive intentions driving our behavior should be a source of relief, because now your weight struggle goes from being a horrible, irrational disease that is happening to you, to a clever strategy you've been using to meet legitimate needs. This is the starting point of healing and sustainable weight loss.

PLEASURE PRACTICE
How Might Your Extra Weight Be Serving You?

Use the Scales of Getting What You Want chart. On the right, list what you hope to get out of losing weight. On the left, list the purposes your extra pounds serve. How have they been helping you feel safe or comfortable? How does the extra weight you are carrying "make sense"? How has it been protecting you? What is the underlying positive intention? Then, ask yourself how else you can honor these positive intentions without needing extra weight to do the job. Is the extra weight needed anymore?

As you imagine letting go of your pattern, which has kept you safe for so long, notice what feelings come up. Do you feel sad, anxious, scared, or depressed? Do you feel tempted to run and binge? These are all natural feelings to have when you are about to let go of a strategy that has been so effective and close to your heart.

The next time you are faced with a craving, instead of reacting automatically based on past decisions that are no longer applicable, listen more deeply and ask yourself, "Where did that choice come from? Is it still relevant or useful? What other options do I have? What would serve me best now?" This opens up a slew of new possibilities, and without pushing, restriction, or denial, you can gradually free yourself from the cravings cycle and establish a new ecology.

APPRECIATING THE PRESENT STATE

Once you've identified the positive intentions that generated your relationship with food and weight, you have the ability to overcome the pull of your old ecology and to create real and lasting change. This secret to pleasurable weight loss is about appreciating the present state. This doesn't mean that you are happy about your circumstances or that you are resigning yourself to your life always being as it is. Instead, it means honoring with compassion your current situation (that is, your current weight) and its well-intended origin, while recognizing your freedom to change it. Transformational coach Stacey Morgenstern says, "There is great power in appreciating the original positive intention of the present state: to protect us, to avoid danger, or to keep us safe. It has served us so well all this time! From this place of appreciation, we can make choices that preserve the positive intention while updating the methods for keeping ourselves safe."

Look into the shadowy corners of your life, where you would rather not look, and ask yourself, "What am I trying to hide, even from myself? What am I hoping others won't know about me?" The answers you come up with will show you where you have shame and where you are in denial of the present state. For example, if you have a hidden daily habit of turning to sugar for a boost, bring it to the surface and let yourself appreciate that this is how it is. You may not be proud of that fact, but for now, you have this habit. In order to get rid of it, you have to own it. It may seem counter-intuitive that the mere act of revealing what is true can change your ecology, but until this appreciation of what is really happening takes place, I have never seen a lasting transformation occur.

Next, in an act of courageous transparency, reveal this shame to someone you trust. One of the secrets to pleasurable weight loss is that once you embrace transparency, your body can relax because you're no longer doing the extra work of hiding who you are. The act of revealing your shame starts to dispel it. Every time I have shared something I was deeply ashamed of, the response from my carefully chosen friends has always lessened my shame. Time and again, my shame has been met with, "You're ashamed of that? That's fairly understandable. It's no big deal." In other words, the cause of my shame always seems worse to me than to others. Relieved of the burden of carrying shame in silence and secrecy, my metabolism instantly benefited once the stress was released.

When you start appreciating the present state, free of shame, you will find you are in a much more powerful and creative position. For example, let's say you've been procrastinating on exercising. You have a gym membership, but you never go. By appreciating the present state, you would move out of denial and into a clear understanding that "I never go to the gym." Now, in the plain light of day, without trying to deceive yourself or anyone else, you are able to return to the question of movement for your body: "I never go to the gym. What would support me in moving my body?" Freed of denial you are also free to brainstorm new solutions.

CONNECTING TO THE NATURAL WORLD

Elie had been a regional manager for Weight Watchers for several years when she rang me in a state of panic. She had risen through the ranks, from member to local leader to manager; she now supervised all the branch leaders in her state. Yet as much as she sincerely tried to embody the method she was endorsing, Elie was eating compulsively and neglecting her points to the degree that she no longer saw any point in keeping count. In public, she tried to give the appearance that she was a model of virtue because she felt her food choices were constantly scrutinized, but when she was alone at home or in her car driving the long distance required for her job, she would binge on chips and sweets.

Elie found me on the Internet, read about my philosophy, and realized that the only weight loss model she hadn't tried was pleasure. As I guided her to investigate her true pleasures, she realized that spending time in nature was what brought her the most delight, even though she rarely made time for it. When she was in nature, Elie felt refreshed, relaxed, stimulated, and open. Her mind came to rest, while her senses came to life. I totally understood Elie's response; connecting to nature is supremely relaxing and healing.

Elie and I worked together to discover new ways to make spending more time in nature a permanent feature of her lifestyle, not just an occasional treat. Her long drive for work gave her many opportunities to pull off the road to a nature reserve, so she began taking walks in the woods alone on weekdays. On the weekends, she'd bring her three kids along.

Making this one simple change to be in nature more had a marked effect on Elie's food cravings and compulsions. As she treated herself to pleasure, she noticed her urge for sweet treats fading away. In public, she felt more confident to eat guided by her appetite, without regard for what anyone else might think about her.

There's nothing like time spent with Mother Nature to bring the wisdom of your female animal to the forefront of your life. When you commune with nature, you realize that you are part of her intricate web and intelligence. You are a feminine creature who is the descendant of a long line of feminine beings, going all the way back to the beginning of life itself. You carry within you a wisdom that has been distilled through the eons. Your body has the power to create life and, therefore, the future. Whether or not you choose to have a child, you are a creator, and as one, this impulse infuses everything you do.

To engage more with the feminine, connecting with nature is an unsurpassed medium. Whether you walk barefoot on grass, enter water, gaze at the stars, smell flowers, or hike, communing with nature reliably relaxes our nervous system. Then we instinctively feel more feminine. Nature connects us with our bodies, grounds us, and makes us more magnetic to others. A woman who is fully connected to the feminine is glorious. When you tune into nature and allow yourself to feel your feminine essence, you create an ecological shift that will change your relationship with your body and with food.

Watch a sunset or a sunrise. Even if you are in the most urban environment, where nature seems far away, as long as the sky is not too cloudy or hazy, the sun, the stars, and the moon are elements of nature you can connect with.

AN ECOLOGY OF ABUNDANCE: OVERCOMING I AM NOT ENOUGH

Women who are struggling with food, weight, and body image share the experience of a haunting inner voice that says, "I'm not enough." I struggled with this for years. I couldn't talk myself out of it, and it plagued me with a deep, shameful knot in my belly. I gave the outside world a facade of self-confidence, but it masked how insecure I really felt. When you feel at your core that you are not enough, you project that lack into other areas of your life. For example, when I felt like I wasn't enough, I also felt I didn't have enough money or time, and I frequently judged my partner for all the ways he wasn't enough, too.

When you perpetually feel insufficient, it puts your body into low-level, chronic stress response, which forces her to hold on to weight. Your feeling of not being enough is translated into not having enough, which sends a physiological signal that real scarcity is at hand. Perceiving a danger to protect against, the body reacts by slowing down the metabolism and holding on to fat reserves. If you then go on to use your extra weight to justify your feeling of inadequacy, you become caught in another infinite shame loop.

The problem is thinking that if we could only lose weight, make more money, or *fill in the blank,* we would then feel enough. This rationalizing never works. There are people who have enormous material wealth but who continue to feel that they do not have enough. There are gorgeous fashion models who don't feel beautiful enough, and brilliant thinkers who don't feel smart enough. And so it goes with scarcity thinking. It's an itch you can never scratch because it's based on a flawed way of thinking. It is based on an ephemeral goal that gets further away from you the closer you move toward it.

I want you to abandon the concept of not being enough altogether, especially when it comes to your weight. The idea of enough is a trap that has no escape. The answer to the questions "Is there enough?" or "Am I enough?" is always no, because it is a question that is not meant to be asked. What's true is that you are enough; you always have been and always will be. There is no external measurement for being enough in this world; either you decide that you are or you stay caught in the illusion that you are not. Only you can decide when you are good enough, sexy enough, or beautiful enough. Again, the truth is that you already are. When you let the background chatter of "there's not enough" or "I'm not enough" fade away, you begin to see that you have enough and that you are enough. When you do, you remove a significant source of chronic stress from your life. This is the foundation for a new ecology of pleasurable weight loss.

THE ECOLOGY OF LOVE, SAFETY, AND BELONGING

Some of the steps for establishing the ideal ecology for weight loss are simple and practical. For example, if not knowing how to cook is holding you back from eating healthy food at home, take cooking classes—you can even learn a lot from the many cooking shows on TV. If eating sugar comforts you at the end of a long day, explore options for different relaxation strategies, including those in the Pleasure Bites. But some of the benefits you are getting from food and weight cannot be addressed like an item on a to-do list. They require a deeper understanding of your psychology to get to the root of what is going on.

Humans have three basic needs—love, safety, and belonging—which developed when we were evolving on the savannas. The need for safety is governed by the basic fight-or-flight response and self-regulation (see Chapter 3). In order to lose weight sustainably, you need to recognize that you are safe and that your needs will be met.

Belonging is the next level of human need. As we evolved, our safety and survival necessitated cooperation within a group or tribe; rejection meant sure death. Our need for connection begins with our family of origin, also known in psychology as a *family system.*

One of the basic tenets of family systems theory is that all parents love their children, and all children love their parents.

There's nothing you can do to be loved any more or any less. Even if your parents were not competent in their demonstration of that love, were even abusive or abandoned you, they still loved you. They were just limited in their capacity because of their own wounds and role models.

The family system encompasses an inheritance that affects us on two levels: genes and memes. The DNA we inherit from our parents determines our genetic code. Our memetic code is made up of our family's beliefs and values. Our parents instill these memes during the first five years of life; with our conscious attention, they can be changed. Although our genetic code can't be changed, the new science of epigenetics teaches us that many genetic tendencies are expressed or repressed depending on environmental factors. Since our beliefs and values are part of our ecology, we know then that our thoughts impact the genetic expression of our DNA. This means that even if you have a genetic potential for obesity, by choosing to create a healthy ecology, you strengthen the possibility of nonetheless being slim.

Our family's beliefs determine what is safe for us to believe about ourselves and our bodies. Before we are even able to talk, we make decisions about how the world works, which become strategies for keeping love, safety, and belonging intact. These beliefs, which are so ingrained we don't question them, become the basis of our patterns. Whatever patterns you have with food and weight are rooted in the beliefs you carry.

We pursue belonging above all, even when it might not be good for us, because we're hardwired to avoid rejection. When we're young, we of course learn through the careful observation and repetition of our parents' behavior. By the time we are old enough to ask our mothers how they feel about their bodies, we have long before interpreted their feelings and likely adopted them. If your mother never liked her hips, it's likely you won't like yours. The same goes for her beliefs about food, sensuality, and pleasure. When you reach a plateau or holding pattern in any area of your life, including weight loss, and there's no apparent reason why you can't break through, it's likely because you would be breaching your family's memetic code. For example, if you want to have a more active lifestyle but can't seem to find the time, it might be because you subconsciously want to stay in rapport with your mother and her relationship, or lack thereof, with movement.

Each family system has its own pros and cons, and to be aware of them gives you a huge advantage when it comes to healing your suffering—and thereby moving from the stress response to a state of relaxation. Each family system's influence tends to go back three generations. For example, if your grandparents lived through food rations, you may have inherited an intense scarcity mentality. The same dynamic among generations also imprints positive attributes. Your grandmother might have become a master gardener in order to put fresh vegetables on the table, which could be why you have a green thumb. So while we can't escape our family system, we can learn from their experiences in order to evolve our own ecology.

The last primary human need is love. The way we learn to show love is tied to belonging. Healthy familial love develops into compassion for others as well as ourselves, but unhealthy family experiences can lead to abuse, addiction, and other forms of suffering. These negative traits get passed down through a process called "the suffering obligation of love," a term first coined by Carl Buchheit, the founder of NLP (Neuro-Linguistic Programming) Marin.

Buchheit describes suffering with our parents as an unworkable effort to let our parents know we love them. Witnessing a parent's suffering, whether it is something trivial and momentary or something chronic, is excruciating for a child. Because children cannot imagine that the cause of their parents' suffering could be anything other than themselves, they identify themselves as the solution to the family's pain. As children, we will do everything we can to try to take away the pain, but try as we may, a child can't eliminate an adult's suffering. Recognizing our failure, we show our allegiance by joining our parents in their suffering, believing that in this way we are reducing the pain because now they are not suffering alone. But this strategy never works: suffering with someone does not make the pain go away.

If your suffering encompasses a bad body image and an unhealthy relationship with food and weight gain, this may well be how you learned to show love to your family. The suffering is your proof that you belong and love your parents—so much so that love becomes indistinguishable from the suffering itself.

Can you see the unworkable ways you have of saying "I love you" to your parents? Here are a few suffering obligations of love you might recognize:

- I will be a victim like you so that you don't feel like a victim alone.
- I will deny my sexuality because you have denied yours.
- I will put myself last and everyone else first, just the way you do.
- I will finish everything on my plate because you think leaving food is a waste.
- I will hate my body because you hate yours.

The way to end a suffering obligation of love is to see the beauty of this misguided positive intention and the absurdity of the method and then to resign your role as the family's solution to pain. Instead, make choices based on what is best for you now, not what allowed you to belong to your family in the past. When you become aware of the suffering obligations you adopted, you become aware of the unnecessary burdens you are carrying, which inevitably weigh you down and make you feel heavy.

When my client Janine came to see me, she lived a largely sedentary lifestyle, ate only rich foods, and never drank a drop of water. When I dug deeper into her story, an interesting fact was revealed. While Janine was growing up, her mother was a smart, driven woman, one of the first female executives in the music business. She prized the power of the mind above all, disdained her own body, and had no interest in exercise. When Janine took up jogging, her mother criticized her saying, "Why would you bother wasting time doing that?" As Janine and I explored her inner ecology, we discovered that when she chose to live a sedentary lifestyle and rejected water as being "too plain" in favor of drinking more "sophisticated" beverages, she felt connected to her mother. She and her mother didn't always have a harmonious relationship, but repeating her mother's choices allowed Janine to feel a connection to her. Once Janine was able to distinguish the influence of the suffering obligation of love in her attitudes toward movement and water, she was able to let go of this strategy for belonging. As her inner ecology changed, she confidently embraced movement, drank water, and lost weight.

Once you realize you can love your parents without having to adopt their burdens, beliefs, and limitations, you are free to relate with them based on your own values. Every time you notice yourself suffering or run up against a perplexing limitation or a pleasure threshold and your first reaction is to criticize yourself, remember that your suffering is your well-intentioned attempt to belong. Instead of continuing to suffer, including any suffering related to food and your weight, say to yourself: "I love you, Mom. I love you, Dad. I know you've suffered a lot. But this is your suffering. Now I'm giving it back to you."

BECOME A FREE WOMAN

If you want to lose weight in a pleasurable way, enjoy a healthy relationship with food, love your body, and feel wonderful about yourself, but these experiences were not part of your family's ecology, then you must learn to relate to your parents in a different way. I spent so many years of my life wishing my mother would understand and approve of me. What I didn't realize was that as long as I was seeking her validation, I was still an adolescent, even though I was well into my adult years. Many of my clients struggle with this same issue of needing their mothers' approval to live the life they want.

It's natural for children and adolescents to need and want their parents' approval. Yet being an adult means expanding beyond your parents' thoughts and beliefs. When you step outside of their ecology, what they understand to be safe, you may well be met with their criticism or disapproval. Their reaction is their instinctive attempt to keep you safe from the unknown. Maybe pleasurable weight loss is a new paradigm that your parents can't support. Your attempts to be happier, slimmer, or sexier may be threatening or unfamiliar to them, but don't interpret their negativity to mean they don't love you. Instead it signifies that you are successfully evolving beyond what they know as true.

For example, my client Paula grew up with a mother who was hyperconcerned with appearances. She imposed a rule never to leave the house without wearing makeup. Even as grown adults, her older sisters conformed, but Paula continues to be chastised by her mother because she never wears makeup. Whenever her mother sees her, she still exclaims, "Who are you not to wear makeup?" The unspoken belief in her mother's ecology is, "The women in this family aren't beautiful enough to go without makeup." As an adult, Paula recognizes that her mother's comments, however hurtful, are an expression of her love, and she wisely chooses to disregard them.

Just as an acorn swept downstream germinates in a microecology different from the one of its mother tree, you have grown up in the unique conditions of your time, which are different from your parents' time. You are the most recent evolution of your lineage. Embrace being different. Don't look back in time for how you are meant to be; look forward. If you're not getting approval from your parents, take it as a sign that you have evolved beyond their worldview. When you can let go of your desire for their approval, you'll find you can go beyond the bounds of your current dreams. Every time I find myself falling back into seeking my parents' validation, I use the following mantra: "I love myself even without your approval." You can also use this mantra with regards to your partner and friends.

Once I realized it is natural to step outside of my mother's ecology, I was able to let go of the disappointment of not having her approval. A huge weight was lifted off my shoulders, and simultaneously a burden was removed from my metabolism. You, too, can put your parents' beliefs aside and begin to live your own life freely, creating a new ecology for pleasurable weight loss and evolving into the amazing woman you were born to be.

PLEASURE PRACTICE
Determining the Beliefs of Your New Ecology

Beliefs form your reality and give the world around you its meaning. You have to become conscious of your family's beliefs, and then choose which are going to serve you and which you can discard. If you are struggling with food and weight, chances are, you carry family beliefs that are not serving you. What are your family's beliefs and rules regarding food, weight, pleasure, and sensuality?

In order to retire beliefs from your ecology that you now recognize are not serving you, you need to import new ones. For example, a valuable belief is to hold the feminine principle in high regard. Another is to believe that you deserve pleasure as a daily nutrient instead of as an occasional reward. A healthy belief about food is that it is a source of nourishment and healing. One way to cement these beliefs is by spending time with others who also value them.

HOW YOU LOVE YOUR MOTHER IS HOW YOU LOVE YOURSELF

Your relationship with your mother sets the tone for your relationship with your body. She represents the feminine side of you. She is where you came from, and you are literally a part of her. When you attack your mother, you attack the feminine side of you, which means, you attack yourself. When you dwell in judgments, anger, or victim stories against your mother, your animal perceives that as a personal attack. Harboring negative feelings toward your mother is also a source of stress. If you are angry or disappointed with her, on some level, you will experience those same feelings toward yourself.

I used to resent many of my mother's attributes until I realized that everything I disdained in her, in some way, I also embodied. I then began the process of letting go of my judgments of her and loving her unconditionally. Once I let go of my judgments toward her, I was able to stop judging those qualities in myself, and I moved into a more open-hearted and compassionate space for both of us.

To heal your relationship with food and your body, it is essential to forgive your mother. Have compassion for her, both now and for the past. Appreciate her not only as your mother but also as an extension of Mother Earth. Take the pressure off of her to fulfill your every dream of what a mother should be. Instead, think of her as a teacher who sometimes led by example and at other times taught you through her mistakes. Let Mother Earth herself, in all her forms and manifestations, be the great mother who guides you and supports you.

Some women have lost their mothers; others have had mothers who were there but did not provide the loving support they needed. Instead of searching for another source of this love, it's time to give it to yourself. Investigate the qualities of love you feel are missing in your life, and then mother yourself in all the ways your mother didn't. If your mother didn't praise you, praise yourself. If she didn't teach you good boundaries, teach yourself. And if you are a mother, access the love you feel for your children and give it to yourself, too.

Meditation teacher Patricia Ellsberg says, "Ironically, the more you need love, the more scarce it is. And the more you can access loving feelings toward yourself, the more the world will rise up to love you." Feeling loved provides relaxation, and it creates the ideal ecology for pleasurable weight loss.

CHANGE YOUR ECOLOGY BY CHANGING YOUR TRIBE

Staying motivated is an expected challenge as you strive to lose weight. As much as we want to move on from where we are, we're all susceptible to the powerful pull of the status quo, which persistently draws us to keep things as they are rather than transform them to something new.

The best way to change your ecology is to change your community. Motivational speaker and author Jim Rohn said that we become the average of the five people we spend most of our time with—in terms of our income, weight, happiness, etc. This means that if the people you most closely associate with hate their bodies and distrust pleasure, then you will, too.

PLEASURE BITE

Host a tea party at your home or a picnic in the park. Expand your inner circle by inviting pleasure-positive friends and ask them to bring someone like-minded along. Enjoy meeting new people.

I was raised in a family that eats really fast, and when I was training myself to eat slowly, I made it a point to eat with friends who I noticed ate slowly. I chose to "belong" with people who believed in the value of eating slowly so that their behavior would rub off on me. This strategy is so effective because of mirror neurons, brain cells that mimic the feelings, actions, and sensations of others. Shawn Achor, author of the *The Happiness Advantage,* points out that mirror neurons explain how we pick up on all emotions, whether they are positive or negative. "Like secondhand smoke, the leakage of emotions can make a bystander an innocent casualty of someone else's toxic state. This means that when we feel anxious or adopt an overtly negative mind-set, these feelings will start to seep into every interaction we have, whether we like it or not."

The fastest way to adopt mind-sets and behaviors that will cause you to lose weight pleasurably is to join a community of women who are already embodying the principles of pleasurable weight loss. This means going to the places they go. Start hanging around women who enjoy their lives, are physically active, buy healthy foods, honor their sensuality, revel in their erotic nature, and deeply honor that they are feminine beings. If your current social circle does not include these types of women, then invest in attending the types of workshops, classes, and events where you will meet them, so that such friendships can be born.

PLEASURABLE EATING PRACTICE 6
Master the Art of Chewing

There is something very relaxing about thoroughly chewing your food, and it also helps you enjoy the whole spectrum of tastes and aromas that make up the meal. I've found that chewing makes food taste better and increases the pleasure of every bite. This is especially true when you are eating whole grains and vegetables, which become sweeter the more they are broken down in the mouth.

Chewing initiates the release of enzymes that allow your body to assimilate more nutrients from the food you eat, prevents gas and bloating, and makes digestion more effi- cient. You may find that when you chew your food more thoroughly your body begins to feel wonderfully light after eating. You'll also be able to better identify the point at which a particular food no longer adds pleasure because you'll be more present.

To master the art of chewing, follow these simple steps. First, place a bite of food in your mouth. Then put down your utensil. Start to chew, and as you do, continue breathing deeply. Close your eyes partly or fully, or focus your gaze on your meal or some other part of your environment that you find relaxing. Take small breaks throughout the meal to slow down the entire experience. Check in with your animal before each new bite to make sure you are still hungry. As you fully chew your food, relish all of the tastes and textures. Let the act of chewing relax you and connect you with your animal instincts.

Darling, I never step on the scale, because the scale doesn't measure sexy.

BELLA DOLCE

7

Until Sexy Is Safe, You'll Never Lose the Weight

WEIGHT AND SEXUALITY are inextricably linked. Whenever I ask a woman why she wants to lose weight, one of the inevitable answers is to feel sexy. It's a perfectly natural desire for every woman to have. It is without question what her female animal wants to feel: sensual and sexual. Yet when I dig a little deeper, I discover another layer within women's psyches that is full of reservations and fears about being sexy.

As much as she wants to embrace her sexual nature, a woman may be wary of the negative ramifications of being a fully embodied sexual woman in our culture. One of the overwhelming patterns I've noticed is a discrepancy between what women say they want when it comes to being sexy and how much sexual energy they are actually comfortable experiencing.

I break the ice on this topic in my live workshops by asking, "When you think about a sexy woman, what single word comes to mind?" I can barely write fast enough on my flipchart to capture all the responses as the words fly in: shallow, bitchy, insecure, intimidating, selfish, manipulative, competitive, man stealer, home wrecker, inauthentic, unprofessional, unearned success, vain, threatening, stupid, airhead, bimbo, and the most derogatory of all, slutty. Next come the judgments and fears: a sexy woman is not a real friend, not a serious person, not smart, is preoccupied with pleasing men, uses her body to get ahead, will abandon her sisters for a guy. All this comes from the same women who only minutes before were telling me they wanted to be sexy!

Women internalize a mixed message about themselves: women are supposed to be sexy, but it's not appropriate for me. On one hand, we are told the quest for beauty and sexiness should be pursued at all costs, and on the other, we are told there is a price to pay for looking too sexy:

- If you look too good, people might overlook your intelligence.
- If you are too attractive, other women will be jealous.
- If you look too hot, you won't be taken seriously.
- If you are too self-assured, you'll be thought of as a bitch.
- If you are too sexy, you are asking to be sexually harassed or assaulted.

Even if you are successfully following a diet and regularly exercising, you'll trigger a low-level chronic stress response (that will cause you to gain weight again) if the idea of being perceived as sexy stresses you out. Until you can embrace yourself as a sexual creature who can fend for herself in a sometimes unsafe world, who can be loved and respected, and who can enjoy herself, your intelligent female animal will make sure you are protected from the danger of your fears by gaining weight. Gaining weight and becoming bigger can be a way to deflect sexual attention. Gain some weight and deflect a little; gain a lot and likely deflect sexual attention altogether.

Most weight loss approaches don't broach this subject, which is another reason why they haven't been working for you. When you lose weight in the feminine, pleasurable way by becoming more attuned to your female animal's needs, you become more sexually attractive before you've even lost a pound. You also learn to handle being more sexually attractive, including all the negative projections that come along with it.

So the next secret to pleasurable weight loss is to learn how to handle the heat of your sexuality and the attention it attracts, so that you can relax into it and let go of the need for the protection of body weight. The more you can embrace a positive and holistic attitude to sexuality, free of guilt or shame—a shift I refer to as becoming sex-positive—the more successful you'll be at losing weight and healing your relationship with food. Then, when welcome sexual attention does come your way, you will be open to receive it.

PLEASURE PRACTICE
Reframing Sexy

Up until now, what have been your negative judgments about sexy women? You may have an elaborate, already formed story about what this type of woman represents. What do you personally fear about being sexy? Think about what would be available to you if you could rise above society's projections and create a new inner and outer ecology about feeling and looking sexy. Let feeling sexy accelerate your pleasurable weight loss.

GETTING PAST THE OLD ECOLOGY
AND THE OBJECTIONS TO SEXY BEING SAFE

Because your subconscious will never allow you to become that which you fear, let's start to unpack your existing ecology for sexuality, including your beliefs about being a sexy woman. Even if you were raised in a liberal family and don't feel that sexual shame was thrust upon you, be aware that the judgments so fully permeate our culture that no woman can avoid being affected by them. Although caught in this struggle between wanting to be sexy and wanting to avoid it at the same time, most women are unaware this inner conflict is sabotaging their weight loss efforts. This stressful schism puts your innocent, sensuous, and sexual female animal into a quandary that promotes weight gain.

Women commonly encounter four main objections when they set out to reframe sexy as safe, and there are four mantras I teach to counter each of these objections. You may have internalized one, two, three, or all of these objections. Once you know how to resolve them within your inner ecology, you can experience being sexy as safe in your life. The mantras below provide you with a practical foundation to make sexy safe, which can be strengthened over time. This deep healing work is often explored at my live Pleasure Camps.

The first objection is always an inner voice that says, "Who am I to be sexy?" If you come from a family system where your mother was sexually repressed or dissatisfied, you may be unconsciously living out a suffering obligation to your mother: "Mom, I will be sexually dissatisfied, so you don't have to be sexually dissatisfied alone." Every woman not only deserves but also needs to access her feminine sexuality in order to maximize her potential in life. One way to begin to quiet the naysaying voice in your head is to use this mantra: "I am a sexual creature, and my sexy is sacred."

The second objection to your own sexiness might be the fear of what other women will think. If you turn on your inner light, then what will your friend/sister/co-worker think of you? Will you be judged as an insatiable woman who willfully disrupts other people's relationships? The mantra to counter a fear that women whose opinions matter to you will be jealous or disapproving is, "I am a mirror of your natural sexy, so let's embody this together."

The third objection comes from a woman's uncertainty about the attention she will receive from those she's attracted to and those who are attracted to her. Even though she wants the attention, she's scared that she won't be able to handle it. If you share this fear, you can work on countering this objection with this mantra: "I am ready to receive your worship. I was born to be adored by you."

The last objection comes from concern about handling the men or women who find you attractive but you don't find attractive in return. How will you say no? For this, you'll use the intimate decline, which you'll learn more about a bit later. The mantra for this objection is, "I appreciate your worship of the feminine, and here's my intimate decline."

PLEASURE PRACTICE
Stepping into the Spotlight

Many women make a conscious effort to hide and down-play their beauty, their radiance, and their sexiness. They fear what others may think about them, and they fear the opportunities and changes that being sexy will create. In what ways do you hide your sexiness? How would your life be different if you were as outwardly sexy as you could be?

YOUR TURN-ON TURNS ON YOUR METABOLISM

Being ashamed of your sexuality can be a source of a chronic stress response that keeps you in a cycle of gaining weight. The opposite is also true. Your turn-on turns on your metabolism. And though the term *turn-on* is mostly used to describe sexual arousal, I am talking about whatever lights you up and ignites you in the broad-est sense. We can also be turned on by food, our career, a rose bush, a sunset, and myriad things that are really meaningful to us. Being turned on, whatever the source, opens and relaxes us, which of course triggers the relaxation response that accelerates weight loss.

One of the great myths about female sexuality—which pre-vents us from maximizing the many benefits of connecting with our turn-on—is that we should feel sexually lit up only in spe-cific sanctioned situations. For example, we've been led to believe that the right time to feel sexual is when we're on a date or in the bedroom with our partner. In most other circumstances, we're told it is wrong or inappropriate. Yet these limitations couldn't be further from the truth. "Our bodies are built to experience turn-on and a level of sexual excitement flowing through us all the time," says women's sexuality expert Layla Martin. "It's a kind of passion you can feel when you're walking down the street, when you're ordering coffee at the coffee shop, when you're at your desk surfing the Internet, that level of turn-on is something so fundamental to your body as a woman, that it's one of the healthiest biological states to be in."

When you cut off the flow of your turn-on, your female animal senses something important is missing. She becomes sad and depleted, and her natural response is to find something else to fill in the gap. And what better substitute than the number-one socially accepted source of pleasure for women—food! If you've been wondering why you feel a constant gnawing sense of hunger in your belly that no amount of food can satisfy, it may be that on the deepest level you're hungry for permission to feel sexually turned on and excited by life all the time. The call of the cookie jar, and the weight gain that comes with it, may be your animal's way of telling you that you are missing what Layla Martin describes as "that constant day-to-day flow of sexual energy through the body."

Earlier I encouraged you to embrace your struggle with weight as an angel leading you to discover deeper truths about yourself. What if your weight gain is not a signal for you to give up feeling sexy but to prioritize feeling sexy all the more? Overcoming the stigma around being a sexy woman requires a fresh look at what sex and sexuality are really all about. It means challenging the perceptions of the mainstream culture and embracing your own self-defined, empowered definition of what it means to be sexy. Our culture reinforces the idea that a woman doesn't even have the right to feel sexy unless she fits into a narrowly prescribed definition.

For example, evolutionary psychologist Geoffrey Miller told me, "I've done enough market research consulting that I know that it's not just a conspiracy theory to say that marketers intentionally try to instill a sense of sexual inadequacy in women in order to be able to offer their products as the cure. Consumerism depends on feeling sexually inadequate. Furthermore, there's no counter-balancing force. Generally, there aren't large companies or political interests that really want women to be satisfied with their sexual desires, their sexual being, or their relationships; because if women have great sex whenever they want with whoever they can seduce, then what else do you want in life? The marketers' worldview is that if everybody had high sexual self-esteem and a healthy self-image, consumers wouldn't bother buying most of what we buy. And they're right."

But even when women embrace their desire to express their sexual nature, many still believe that they have to lose weight first. And because not feeling sexy is a stressor that you now know makes weight loss difficult, this is a vicious cycle that can prevent you from ever feeling sexy and losing the weight if you do not reverse this loop. Your animal is a sexual creature who is meant to feel sexy and desired, and if your conscious mind is not respectful of her needs, the loss will register as a source of stress.

In Pleasurable Weight Loss, we discard messages from the outside world that tell us we have to wait until we lose weight to feel sexy. The secret is simple: once you recognize how attractive you are and use your sexual energy effectively (instead of hiding it, downplaying it, or neutralizing it), then getting what you want in life becomes a lot easier. Imagine being able to spring out of bed feeling genuinely sensual, sexy, and safe. If you were capable of maintaining those feelings all day, it would put you into a stable state of relaxation—the coveted metabolic state for pleasurable weight loss. Imagine how much more confident and enthusiastic you'd feel in every pursuit of your day then!

My definition of sexy is being united with your primal sexual nature, exuding it, and enjoying it. It is not conforming to what the women's or men's magazines tell you being sexy is supposed to look like. It doesn't carry inauthentic undertones; in fact, it is the authentic expression of who you are. The media stereotypes that reduce sexy to either a porn star or an androgynous sixteen-year-old girl are pervasive, but they're the smallest representation of what being sexy fully encompasses. If you judge your sexiness by those standards, you are doomed to fall short and continue living in the stress response. The secret is to start experiencing yourself as a sexy woman right now. Even if you think your butt is too fat, your belly is too round, your breasts are too small, or your thighs are too big, when you are in touch with the sexual pulse that animates you and all life, you are sexy.

PLEASURABLE EATING PRACTICE 7
Eat Slowly and Sensually

Slow eating invites sensuality and presence. When you eat slowly, it allows you to derive more sensory pleasure from the experience, and because you receive more enjoyment from eating, you are satisfied sooner and ready to put down the fork, without it being a discipline to stop.

Our Western culture and ecology is obsessed with speed, but your animal must eat slowly to attain pleasurable weight loss. Slowing down your eating speed is one of the most important factors for healing emotional eating. When you eat emotionally, you're not present to the taste or the quantity of what you are eating. Eating slowly supports your animal to let you know when she has had enough to eat—cues you otherwise miss out on if you are eating moderately or fast. Your meal can become a valuable occasion to be with your animal, not a utilitarian task to be rushed through.

Eating fast is a stressor unto itself: it's stressful for the body to have to digest food so quickly. As I mentioned before, if you eat too fast, your animal says, "I didn't taste anything, see anything, smell anything, or experience anything," and your brain thinks, "I must still be hungry," making you eat more. When you eat slower, you metabolize faster. Your animal gets more pleasure from the experience and responds by generating a more powerful metabolic response to the meal, enhancing calorie-burning efficiency.

Because eating slowly helps you eat less without feeling in the slightest way deprived, it is one of the secrets of pleasurable weight loss. Consciously allow more time for your snacks and meals, and enjoy the sensual pleasure of eating slowly. Check in with your animal with each bite to make sure you are still hungry.

YOU ARE ALREADY SEXY

One of the very natural reasons we want to feel sexy is we want to attract sexual attention. Though you may think you have to be thin to be the object of sexual desire, you have a distorted view of what men are really attracted to. Evolutionary psychologist Geoffrey Miller explains: "There's a lot of evidence to show that men want women to be a bit plumper and to have more muscle mass than women think. Men's attraction to these characteristics is founded in an evolutionary instinct to choose a strong, fertile woman who can give birth to bigger-brained babies, forage for food more effectively, and be generally capable and healthy.

And remember that most men find most women at least some-what sexually attractive. So today, when a man is looking at a woman, even if she's 'overweight' by her standards—or media standards—he will likely find her more sexually appealing than she thinks he will." Relationship expert Michaela Boehm also reminds us, "The truth of the matter is, a naked body against another naked body always feels good. Women need to under-stand that for most men any naked woman is a beautiful woman."

Even though we've been conditioned to believe that sex is wrong, from an evolutionary perspective, sex has been our *raison d'être*. I want you to find confidence in knowing that every aspect of your physique has been refined through evolution to make you sexually desirable. You come from an unbroken line of highly successful mating creatures. Your entire body is sensual, every part designed for pleasure. The reason women have breasts, a round ass, and thigh fat is that these traits have been turning men and women on for thousands of generations.

Cultivating a feminine aesthetic is another element of feeling sexy. For at least a hundred thousand years, women have been decorating themselves with pigments, and for at least forty thou-sand years, women have been adorning themselves with jewelry. So remember that when you feel like getting dressed up, you're not just conforming to the fashion industry's standards but also participating in an authentic evolutionary expression women have enjoyed to enhance their sexual appeal, long before fashion magazines ever existed.

Some of the sexiest women I've seen are not slender and lean, but they carry themselves with grace and confidence. It's not only your body that constitutes your sex appeal. Your humor, your language skills, your self-confidence, your social skills, your success, your taste, your style, your charm, and your grace are all sexy qualities that you can possess at any weight. Sex expert Alex Allman says, "In my study of thousands of men about what they most craved from a woman during sex, more than anything else, was a woman who had a positive and comfortable relationship with her own body and sexuality. In a culture designed to make women feel insecure about their bodies, it's no surprise that men seem to find this experience excruciatingly rare."

PLEASURE PRACTICE
Defining Sexy for You

Even if your inner ecology of thoughts, beliefs, and values has been conditioned to distrust sex, your animal knows a deeper truth. Your ideas about becoming sexy need to feel in alignment with who you are at every level—mentally, emotionally, physically, and spiritually—without contradiction in order for you to fully achieve it. You'll need to examine all of these aspects of your ecology to see what new beliefs need to be created to make your whole life congruent.

Define what makes you feel sexy. Complete the sentence "I feel sexy when . . . " with as many possibilities as you can think of. Which people and which environments encourage you to feel sexy? What clothes make you feel sexy? What mood, what music, what frame of mind makes you feel sexy? What does being sexy mean to you? Create a definition of sexy that you can embody right now.

YOUR PRIMAL HUNGER

The longing for food and sex are two primal hungers, the relationship between which is undeniable: both are forces beyond our conscious control that demand our appreciation and understanding. Your animal already knows that it's perfectly natural to have an appetite, be it for food or sex or anything. Yet women are often scared of their hunger for food and sex. The truth is, we are born with hunger and desire, so it is important to make peace with this so that we can release any shame and guilt we may feel about our desires.

If you've been struggling with endless food cravings and the size of your appetite, these may be symptoms of sexual dissatisfaction. Sexual pleasure is a requirement of a healthy life and a happy female animal. It's not enough just to go through the motions of having sex. You have to be fully engaged to maximize your satisfaction. So the next time you find yourself cranky and grumpy and your inclination is to eat to feel better, a mind-blowing orgasm might be exactly what you need!

Orgasms are a biological imperative. They stimulate the brain in a very specific way, releasing a host of biochemical reactions, one of the most notable being the generation of dopamine. Anything that brings us pleasure releases dopamine. That's why when you experience an orgasm, you can rewire your brain's reward circuitry to replace the compulsive search for sugar with something much more beneficial for your animal—and a lot more fun.

"Dopamine is the ultimate feminist chemical in the female brain," writes Naomi Wolf in *Vagina: A New Biography.* "When a woman's dopamine system is optimally activated—as it is in the anticipation of great sex, an effect heightened by a woman knowing what turns her on, letting herself think about it, and letting herself go get it—it strengthens her sense of focus and motivation levels and energizes her in setting goals. All those effects are involved with dopamine activation. It is accurate to say that if you activate your dopamine system in seeking out great sex that you can take those heightened capabilities of energy and focus into other areas of your life and into other endeavors."

Whereas low dopamine levels correspond with low libido and low energy, by having orgasms, and potentially a multitude of them, maintaining a high level of dopamine allows a woman to be more confident, creative, and sociable. It heightens our sense of independence and the impulse to seek freedom from a grounded basis of self-love. Optimal dopamine levels help a woman to be a decisive leader, for she can be more assertive, express strong opinions, and set clear boundaries. "Great sex makes women hard to push around," writes Naomi Wolf. "If a woman has optimal levels of dopamine, she is difficult to direct against herself. She is hard to drive to self-destruction, to manipulate and control." All the more so for a woman who is very orgasmic. Balancing brain chemistry through orgasms also provides a calm feeling of well-being and satisfaction and makes life feel more meaningful.

The secret to pleasurable weight loss is always to put your pleasure first—and not to wait until you lose weight. Therefore, you must prioritize sexual pleasure in your life. If you already have a rockin' sex life, good for you! Expand your horizons all the more. And if you don't, now is the time to realize the importance of sexual pleasure. Missing out on sex is like missing out on an essential nutrient in your diet—deep down you will always feel deprived.

When I ask women how well they are feeding their sexual appetite, I frequently get the same response: "I don't have much of a sexual appetite anymore, and I don't particularly care." If you don't believe that you deserve to feel sexy, you'll tune out the stirrings of your sexual appetite, and because you stop listening to your female animal's true desires, she gets tired of being ignored and her cry for erotic fulfillment gets reduced to a whimper. If you've stopped feeling sexy, it's because you've stopped paying attention.

Only you can know your desires. But many women often loathe even admitting their desires. I remember that as a teenager I literally cursed them. My experience taught me that my desires only got me into trouble. They compelled me to overeat, and they compelled me to be sexual in ways that my mother did not approve of. I begged my desires to leave me alone so I could get on with being productive, but nothing would make those damned desires go away. Because we have such a culturally fearful relationship with desire, it is easy to fall into the trap of ignoring your desires yet feel dominated by them, causing further stress.

Women shy away from the potential disappointment of not fulfilling their desires by denying them at the outset. If they are afraid that they can't attain the object of their desire, they won't allow themselves to linger in the uncertainty of wanting. I suggest that instead you begin to enjoy exploring your secret desires. The secret is to allow yourself to derive satisfaction from your yearning, distinct from its fulfillment. It's a delicate balance between loving what you have right now and desiring something else. Your desire, even if you don't know how you're going to fulfill it, can be a source of pleasure. You can enjoy wanting to have a delicious lover even before you have one. In this way, you'll also be able to take pleasure in wanting to lose weight, and the process itself will become enjoyable.

While there are countless factors that contribute to an urge to binge or overeat, undiagnosed sexual fulfillment is definitely one of them. "Sexual anorexia" often goes hand in hand with emotional overeating, which compensates for the missed pleasure. Even if you pamper and pleasure yourself with clothes, massages, vacations, and fine dining, you will not feel fully satisfied if your sexual hunger is not met. And your brain can easily confuse this message with the need to eat. The more sexually satisfied you are, the less vulnerable you are to using food, alcohol, shopping, etc., to satisfy your need. When you are free to want what you want without shame, you are congruent within yourself, and your desires will be easier to enjoy and fulfill.

A woman who embraces her desires is irresistible and attractive. Answer the call of your sexual appetite, fully, as you are right now, and seek out and receive the juicy, delicious ravishing your female animal naturally craves.

My client Amelia came to see me because she had been dealing with emotional eating for years. She told me it became more of an issue after she broke up with her partner. Amelia said that during the day she was able to make food choices that supported her weight loss, but come night she was plagued by food cravings. Living in New York City, it was easy for her to order in something sweet, like a piece of chocolate cake or a milkshake, along with something savory.

I guided Amelia to explore how her cravings might be a symptom of other forms of pleasure she was missing out on. Slightly embarrassed, she admitted that when the cutest delivery guys came to her door, she was surprised by the primal urge to get close to them. Amelia realized that her late-night cravings weren't truly about food; they were indicators of her neglected sensual and sexual appetite. Since her breakup, she had replaced real affection and intimacy with chocolate cake. I coached her to turn her attention to proactively meeting new people and dating, and once she did, she reported that she was no longer overeating at home alone. Happily, her animal was being fed in other ways.

PLEASURE PRACTICE
Feed Your Sexual Appetite

If you feel your sexual appetite is diminished or if you simply want to stoke that fire, here are some steps to be more in touch with your potent female libido. Use your mind to help your body feel safe and to express her sexual longings. Talk to your animal and let her know it's safe to have a sexual appetite and to be sexual. You can try affirmations like these:

- I honor your sexual desire.
- Your sexual appetite is welcome.
- Let yourself have the pleasure you were born to enjoy.

SEXUAL NOURISHMENT:
THERE IS MORE PLEASURE THAN YOU KNOW

We used to think that the most important way to measure food was by its caloric content, but today we know that not all calories are created equal and that the quality of food matters, which is why a green juice is always a better choice than a diet soda. Our culture is focused on a calorie-counting equivalent when it comes to sex as well: there's a focus on how long you spend having sex and on how many and what types of orgasms you have.

Layla Martin teaches us to cultivate a more nourishing sexuality: "Nourishing sex has a lot to do with your intention or mind-set, how you feel about your sexuality, and how you feel about your orgasm. Are you only playing the part of having an orgasm or are you, either with your partner or with yourself, connecting intimately and vulnerably and welcoming the full breadth of your emotions, including allowing yourself to cry if you need to cry."

If you are bringing your guilt or shame into the bedroom, thinking, "I'm not pretty enough, I'm not good enough, I'm too fat," then you're not going to have the fulfilling experience that will allow sex to feed your soul at the deepest levels. However, if you can let go of the shame and guilt, let loose, and fully enjoy your female animal the way she was meant to be enjoyed, then your orgasmic energy can literally and metaphorically feed you. It will help end compulsive eating and your struggle with weight. After truly nourishing sex, it feels like all is right in the world.

Once you are free of the shame, you can take your sexual nourishment to the next level. Most of us reach adulthood and are still sexually illiterate. I know I was. I didn't know the name of my clitoris until several years after I started having sex, and it wasn't until recently that I learned the full extent of my pelvic neural network. We have so many different nerve pathways that go through a whole network of structures, including the vagina and other pelvic organs. Because of this, there are multiple kinds of orgasms a woman can have. Orgasms can be expansive and explosive or soft, deep, and oceanic. In fact, there are so many that it can take a happy lifetime of exploration to discover them.

Your sexual energy can also be healing in your efforts to expand your pleasure threshold and experience of relaxation. As you explore your own edges, you can increase your sensations for pleasure beyond your wildest imagination. As an added bonus, you heighten your calorie-burning efficiency and find nourishment other than food.

Because sexual nourishment is a secret to pleasurable weight loss, I want you to feel empowered to access this source of pleasure all by yourself. Self-pleasuring is so taboo in our society, especially for women, that we often feel our sexual gratification depends on someone else doing it for us, but this doesn't have to be the case. Some women don't have partners, and all of us find ourselves alone at one point or another. Whatever the circumstances, once you learn how, you can deeply pleasure and satisfy yourself. Although our culture leads us to believe that self-pleasuring is a dirty habit and certainly a poor substitute for "the real thing," which is having sex with someone else, sex educator Betty Dodson, author of *Sex for One,* turned my thinking around on this matter. She thinks of self-pleasuring as "solo-sex" and a genuine form of sex unto itself. Regardless of whether I'm in a relationship, now I continue to discover greater pleasure thresholds and subtleties as the years go by. Feeling confident that you can be the source of your own erotic pleasure will boost your self-esteem, and giving that pleasure to yourself counteracts the weight-gaining effects of stress in your world.

EMBRACING YOUR EROTIC INNOCENCE

Your sexuality is fundamentally innocent. The root of the word *erotic* is *Eros,* which comes from the Greek and refers to "that which animates life." If we understand erotic in this context, then it is impossible to segregate it to any one area of the body or mind because Eros imbues everything; it's inherent in the matrix of life. The term *erotic innocence,* coined by Saida Désilets, beautifully puts words to something I always felt deep in my bones. She describes erotic innocence as "undomesticated Eros," which is the unconditioned response of your animal to anything in life that triggers aliveness and, therefore, pleasure.

Your erotic innocence is your female animal's innate impulse toward all that gives you delight, including the sensual, the sexual, and the erotic. Erotic innocence is prelingual and sensory and stems from your reptilian brain. It is innocent because it arises from the most primitive part of you, which existed long before the judging mind evolved to deem these desires right or wrong. Seen through the lens of erotic innocence, your reactions to any form of pleasure are instinctive and a direct response to your immediate experience. Being in touch with the innocent nature of your desire will help you release shame and invite more pleasure into your life.

When you are in touch with your erotic innocence, you will walk through life being guided by what delights and opens your senses. You will experience pleasure everywhere you go, and because of this, you won't have a pleasure deficiency making you vulnerable to overeating and gaining weight. That's why I like to emphasize that the secret to weight loss is not about eating less and exercising more, as the mainstream would have it, but rather about cultivating your erotic innocence. There is no judgment of good or bad when you experience the world through your erotic innocence. Imagine how sexually freeing it would be to have all your mind's judgments quieted so that you could directly hear your body's yearnings.

Your erotic innocence responds to every dimension of life. You could be walking in a forest and be aroused by the curve of a tree. Erotic innocence revels in pleasure and sensuality without a shred of guilt or shame. It is acutely in touch with what feels good and what doesn't. And when you are connected with your erotic innocence, the notion that "you don't know what you want" evaporates, as you are always able to know what you prefer in a given moment. When you allow your erotic innocence to guide you in the world, your experience of the world is transformed, as you are continuously led from one small delight in life to another. Being "turned on" simply becomes another version of "being alive."

Being in touch with the innocent nature at the root of desire is critical for releasing your shame about desire, as well as for feeling safe with another's desire. Connecting with the guiltless, shameless nature of your erotic innocence allows you to reclaim your sexy as safe. And as you do, you invite your body into the relaxed state in which calories burn efficiently and weight loss is a pleasurable side effect.

When my client Diana came to me, she was seeking my help to lose thirty pounds. Raised in a conservative, church-going family, she always wanted to be "cute" but not sexy, so she'd never thought of herself that way. That is, until she met Harry at a business convention. Harry thought Diana was exquisite and desirable, inside and out, and as they got to know each other, they became lovers. Diana had never been adored and desired like this before. I helped her to let go of her shame surrounding sex and taught her to embrace her erotic innocence. Soon her sense of self transformed, and Diana began to think, "I can be sexy; in fact, I want to be sexy." Without trying, she dropped thirty pounds as she released the barrier she'd put between herself and the possibility that she was indeed sexy.

Saida Désilets teaches that the lens of erotic innocence is complemented by a progressive development of erotic wisdom and erotic intelligence. Erotic wisdom helps you create context by taking your emotions and social conditioning into account. With erotic wisdom, you will be able to see where your actions lead so that you can make an informed choice, and not repeat previous mistakes. Erotic intelligence is informed by your life energy but filtered through the mind so that you make rational decisions about your safety and pursuit of pleasure. When you have a healthy relationship among your erotic innocence, erotic wisdom, and erotic intelligence, they work together to provide you with a broader and safer erotic experience.

If you want to live in a world where it is safe to fully express your erotic innocence, it is up to you to tap into communities that are on the same wavelength. Any environment that allows you to be fully congruent, so that you can embody what you feel, is fantastic and will help you learn that it is safe to be your sexy self. Getting together with supportive, nurturing women is a great way to cultivate community. This can be in your home, at parties, at events, or simply while enjoying an evening together. Group activities that are built around an honest appreciation of the feminine—such as tango dancing, salsa dancing, and belly dancing—form their own communities.

There may be situations where being outwardly sexy is dangerous, but that doesn't mean you need to shut down your sexuality completely. If you shut it down all day, every day, then you risk losing the ability to access it. So the secret is never to shut it down; cloak it as needed instead. Then you can turn the dial up or down on your sexual energy as you choose.

PLEASURE BITE

Cultivate your erotic innocence by traveling through the world with an openness and willingness to receive pleasure everywhere you go. With a fresh awareness, follow where your curious erotic innocence leads.

EMBRACE THE ATTENTION

When you become a fully open, sensual, juicy woman, exuding her energy of pleasure in the world, you are going to attract attention. A secret of pleasurable weight loss is being ready and equipped to receive this attention, from both men and women, so that it doesn't cause you stress.

In our culture, the instinctive pull of the polarizing qualities of masculine and feminine has become completely distorted. In *The Way of the Superior Man,* David Deida writes, "Our culture reduces attraction to a sexual thing, whereas it is actually a whole body transmission of energy, affecting the heart as much as, or more, than the genitals. In other cultures, women were honored for their gift of spiritual rejuvenation, not just ogled for sexual titillation." In the modern world, boys and men haven't been trained this way; instead, their understanding of sexuality is heavily influenced by misogynistic cultural norms, including pornography, violent movies, and video games, which distort their perception of how men treat women and justify relationships based on power, domination, and intimidation. Unfortunately, most men are not aware that they retain in their DNA an elemental reverence for the divine feminine, nor are they aware of their responsibility as ambassadors of the divine masculine to honor women and treat them respectfully. This is why I believe that at the root of every catcall and inappropriate remark or gesture a man makes toward a woman is a subconscious deep yearning to worship and be nourished by her feminine energy. This perspective allows compassion for men, and because compassion is a relaxing state, a compassionate perspective supports weight loss.

The more radiant you become, the more you have to learn how to handle and receive all flavors of attention, from gushing compliments to off-color remarks. If you are already comfortable with receiving attention, hallelujah! I'm thrilled to hear it. Thanks for being a role model, showing women how this can be done in a grounded and centered way. But if you find male attention disturbing, then the stress from receiving attention may sabotage your weight loss plans.

One of the most useful ways I've found to stop being triggered or annoyed by catcalls or offensive comments is to imagine that I am translating this crassness through the portal of my heart to reveal its essence, which I believe is always, "I want to be nourished by your feminine energy; I want to worship you." When you can do this, you can reframe any comment as a positive intention and thereby prevent yourself from being triggered into a stress response. This is another example of authoring your reality: create a story about what is going on that better serves you and your pleasurable weight loss goal.

Another inevitable side effect of receiving attention is that it intensifies your sensations. For example, when you are speaking in public, the sensations in your body can become so intense that some people equate their fear of public speaking with their fear of dying. I remember the first time I went on television, I threw up before I went on air, a reaction to the intensity of merely anticipating the attention that would come from being on TV. But if you expect sensation to increase because of attention, then when it comes your way, whether because you are speaking to a large crowd from a podium, or because you are getting more compliments about your legs than you've ever had before, you will be better equipped to handle it. The secret is to stay present and grounded and to let the sensation wash through you, knowing that if you surrender to it, it will soon pass.

You can also channel the intensity of the sensation of attention into other passions and pursuits. Jennifer Russell recommends thinking of your body as a satellite dish that catches all the attention that comes its way and then focuses it into a powerful beam of energy directed to a particular use.

Receiving attention comfortably is like a muscle that grows with practice. At first the sensations may overwhelm, but the more you practice, the more comfortable you will become. The most important thing to remember is that although someone's attention creates a sensation in your body, you have no obligation to respond in any way other than what is authentic for you. You are completely free to act in a way that's true for you and your animal. Do not oblige yourself to fulfill anyone else's agenda. If you are driven by a willingness to please others at your own expense, then your animal will not feel safe because you have demonstrated that you will betray her needs in favor of others.

Once a woman feels comfortable receiving attention and responding authentically, she will no longer be scared of sexual attention. She can then relax into her naturally sexual female body, and in doing so, create within herself the response that leads to weight loss.

PLEASURE BITE

The more pleasure you have in your life, the better you'll look and feel and the more people will notice and comment. Practice receiving compliments gracefully. Say "thank you" with a smile, instead of defensively deflecting the attention away. You deserve to be complimented.

THE INTIMATE DECLINE

Another aspect of becoming comfortable with attention is the ability to set healthy boundaries. For many women, saying no to anything is difficult, and saying no to sexual advances can be that much more difficult. Women are conditioned from a young age to suppress their authentic "no." We're taught to overlook our own desires and to say "yes" to the needs of others. If you don't know how to refuse a sexual advance, then you may be afraid of even the subtlest sexual attention. However, it is possible to enjoy receiving sexual attention while also setting strong, clear boundaries.

I used to be terrible at setting sexual boundaries. I would hear a "no" in my mind but feel too scared to open my mouth and express it for fear of making the other person uncomfortable. So I would swallow my no and submissively go along and do things I didn't want to do. Eventually, I reached a point where I became unwilling to put my female animal in a situation in which she was not relaxed and at ease. I finally learned to say no.

If you habitually say yes when you mean no or constantly bite your tongue and tolerate situations that make you uncomfortable, it's fair to say you have poor boundaries. You avoid saying no in order to stay in others' good graces. But without boundaries, you are unknowingly creating toxic relationships filled with resentment. If you don't know how to say no, you probably feel offended or rejected when other people say no to you.

Saying yes when you mean no has negative consequences. When you are afraid that others won't be able to handle hearing no, you are unconsciously assuming that they need some sort of protection because they are incapable of dealing with your truth. You are undermining their ability to have a reasonable reaction, which includes the freedom to react with compassion or curiosity as much as it does being offended or hurt. So when you begrudgingly go along with plans because you don't want to be rude, you're not only putting yourself in a situation you don't want to be in but also not allowing everyone else to get to know the authentic you or to show more of who they are.

One of the little-known costs of ignoring your no is that others pick up on your betrayal of your boundaries. You are then perceived as less trustworthy and more vulnerable because your personal boundaries are flimsy. Living with poor boundaries is stressful and, therefore, interferes with your ability to lose weight. To make matters worse, when you are stewing in resentment and feeling powerless to do anything about it, you are more likely to overeat in order to numb out the painful feelings—and so the infinite stress loop goes round and round. Instead of putting themselves in a situation where they might feel pressured to do something sexually that they don't want to do, some women will unconsciously use the protection of excess weight to deflect sexual attention. This weight communicates a broad sweeping message of "I'm not sexually available."

If you want to experience lasting, pleasurable weight loss, healthy boundaries are essential. The secret is to feel calm and confident asserting your boundaries. Then you can let your light shine brightly without fear, welcome the attention you want, and deflect the attention you don't want. The simplest formula for acknowledging what you want is to operate from the understanding that if your immediate answer to a question is not yes, then it's a no. Observe your reactions through this lens and start to become more aware of when you truly mean yes or when you are saying yes but your honest response is no. A true yes is easy to recognize because you experience yourself physically moving closer to whatever is in question. Notice too when your body and mind respond differently. Let your mind follow your animal's lead.

Once you are clear about what you want, one of the most powerful ways to create healthy boundaries stems from the martial arts tradition of aikido. It is called the *intimate decline.* The intimate decline is an energetic stance that supports saying no. It is intimate because it acknowledges the desire of another, but at the same time it communicates a firm decline to the request. You are acknowledging that it is fine for another to want what he or she wants, just as it is equally fine for you not to want it.

Let's say a guy you have no interest in starts talking to you at the supermarket and asks you to meet him for coffee. Without the intimate decline, saying no might make you feel flustered, upset, or offended, triggering a stress response. However, if you were to respond with the stance of an intimate decline, you would appreciate the fact that this guy wants to spend time with you and feel equally comfortable communicating no to him directly. The underlying message of such a no would be, "Your desire, although fine for you, is not a match for me." The intimate decline allows you to keep your physiology in the optimal relaxation state.

My client Hannah was a beautiful woman with a voluptuous figure. Hannah told me that when she walked through the streets, she constantly received catcalls. She found them degrading and stressful. The same day I taught her the intimate decline, a man on the street yelled after her, "You're beautiful! Will you marry me?" This time, instead of allowing her blood pressure to rise, Hannah embodied the intimate decline, and she was able to smile at the offer and peacefully walk by.

Setting healthy boundaries is habit forming. The more you honor yourself and others, the more you'll find yourself naturally honoring the needs of your body with healthy food, enjoyable movement, and an array of other pleasures. As pleasure becomes a bigger part of your life, you'll find you will receive more offers than you want to accept. But because you feel proficient with the intimate decline, you will feel safe having your beauty, sensuality, and sexual magnetism for the world to see. You'll know that you can say yes or no as you please to the attention that comes your way. You will feel confident communicating your boundaries, and before long, you'll have the courage to flirt, to wear a short dress, and to be as sexy as you want to be. Once you feel this security and are no longer scared of sexual attention, you will be able to relax deeply into your sexual female body.

Lastly, when you can confidently say no, your yes becomes trustworthy and powerful. It allows others to relax in the assurance that you will represent your needs and wants. Similarly, when you hear a no from others, instead of interpreting it as a rejection, you will be able to thank them for clearly communicating their boundaries.

PLEASURE PRACTICE
Recognize Your Boundaries

Unless you can say no, you can't maintain a relaxed state, and the stress that accompanies your boundaries being crossed will prevent you from losing weight. If you are uncomfortable saying no, make a list of how this affects your life. Then, experiment leaning into the discomfort of expressing your boundaries. You can use responses such as, "That's not a match for me," "I don't feel like it," or "I need some privacy and alone time." Pay attention to the little resentments that build up when you cross your internal boundary, and recognize that every one of them contributes to keeping unwanted weight on your body. Take every opportunity to dissolve these resentments by respecting your healthy boundaries and expressing yourself.

HEALING SEXUAL TRAUMA

A staggering number of women have experienced the trauma of having their sexual boundaries crossed. If not you, it might have been your mother, sister, or a friend. This trauma affects the way a woman views her body, her sexuality, how safe she feels in the world, and, therefore, her relationship with her weight and food.

I know this firsthand because I have experienced sexual trauma. When I was fifteen years old and still a virgin, a boy I had just met at a nightclub raped me on the street. I begged him to stop, but he held me down and penetrated me. I froze. I didn't even scream. My body went limp. When he was done, he pulled down my dress and went on his way. Afterward, the only way I knew to cope with the trauma was to repress the experience. I didn't tell anyone, and I tried my best to block the memory from my mind.

It wasn't until I was nineteen, when I started studying yoga and learned to feel more deeply and be present that the memory of the rape came flooding back. I allowed myself to feel the anger toward this rapist that I'd repressed. I was seething, but I was able to remain present with my pain, rage, and anguish. I faced the agony of my lost innocence and the injustice of someone else's sexuality being forced upon me.

I took time with the healing process. I retreated to my friend Gum's house in the safety of the rainforest where I could scream and cry an ocean of tears. I embraced transparency, one of the secrets of pleasurable weight loss and one of the most powerful tools for healing shame. I began to tell my story to everyone who mattered to me. In the telling and in the presence of their compassionate listening, I began to heal. I sought professional counseling and worked through a book of exercises on healing sexual trauma. I spent as much time as I could in nature, and I continued to practice yoga.

Still, I couldn't let go of the fear that it could happen again. Then one day, as clichéd as it sounds, I heard a voice from the sky clearly say, "You will never be raped again." Simple as that. No explanation. I sighed with relief.

Through my daily yoga practice I became stronger, more confident, more powerful, and I felt safer. I had my wits about me. Nobody would trespass my body again. One Saturday morning when I was twenty, I went to a public beach by myself in the tropical paradise of Martinique, where I was living. Eager to swim in the azure waters, I placed my gear at the edge of the bushes that lined the beach and swam to my heart's content. When I got out of the water and went to find my belongings, a tall, muscular, and naked island man with an enormous erection came charging at me. He grabbed me and threw me on the ground. In that moment, I remembered the voice from the sky that had given me so much comfort: "You will never be raped again." I was determined this would be so. Instead of shutting down and freezing the way I did the last time, I became fully present and started screaming with all the lung power I could muster. Over and over, I screamed, "Help!" I did everything I could to fight. I pulled his hair, and I tried to poke his eyes and kick his groin. He punched me above my eye and blood spilled down my face. I was losing the fight, but I kept screaming, hoping someone would hear me. I kept running the words through my head: "I will not be raped. I will not be raped." My assailant had just succeeded in taking off my bathing suit and was literally inches away from penetrating me when another man came running toward us in response to my screams. The rapist dropped me, ran away, and I never saw him again.

I had saved myself. Between fighting back and my screams, which brought help, I had prevented myself from being raped. In the aftermath, I was just as traumatized as the first time, yet I was better equipped to handle what had happened. Without repressing the experience, I processed the painful emotions to the best of my ability. I soothed my fear by singing simple songs, a way to regulate my nervous system. I continued practicing yoga and meditation every day, and I started learning Afro-Caribbean dancing. I felt a new depth of connection to my body, a playful joy I had never felt before. But I couldn't stop myself from overeating, and I gained twenty pounds.

Through my experiences I came to understand that sometimes the world is not a safe place. Things happen that we don't want to happen. They aren't our fault. Ultimately, we can heal and rise above our traumas. I also learned that if I was going to be safe, I had to be aware and present and take responsibility for setting boundaries and protecting myself. And I learned that even though my innocence had been stolen, I could reclaim it. Coming out of my healing process I had a new sense of feeling whole. This has led me to think of myself as a healer. All these years later, I can see that the root of my confidence in my offerings to the world stems from these traumatic experiences and how I overcame them. For this reason, I can even be grateful for what happened and forgive my perpetrators.

When you have a trauma or abuse in your history, it's an understandable response to soothe your pain with food. Up until now, you may have needed food to feel better and to feel safe. But there are more appropriate ways to meet these needs so that food can return to its natural role as nourishment for your animal. The lessons throughout this book will help you remove the shame and restore your sense of personal power so that you can deal with your feelings as they present themselves. All of these skills will help you through the healing process and make you a more resilient woman.

Until you understand and accept that being a sexual woman can be safe, you'll never lose weight, no matter how much you claim it's what you want. What I've discovered over the years of helping women lose weight is that when they can come to peace and reconciliation with their traumatic past, they no longer sabotage their weight loss or subconsciously avoid expressing their sexuality. Healing is always possible.

SEX IS SACRED

I first encountered the idea that sex is sacred when I went to India. I walked into a small, out-of-the-way temple, and in the center was a large marble statue that looked like a stylized penis, known in Sanskrit as a *lingam,* coming out of a stylized vagina, or *yoni.* Hanging above the sculpture was a copper vessel full of water with a small hole in the bottom that released one drop of water at a time over the phallus, over the yoni, and eventually into a hole on the temple floor. Flowers and incense covered the altar, and the local people came in bowing and saying prayers. I stood there with my jaw practically hitting the ground because I had never seen anything like this in my life. To my eyes it was extremely sensual and erotic to be worshipping this moist and dripping statue. Without any explanation or further knowledge of Hinduism, I got the point: sex and sexuality are sacred.

In the West, we've been conditioned to think divine love is a religious experience achieved by transcending the body, and that the body itself is an obstacle to spirituality. Unlike ancient cultures with archetypes that glorified sexuality as an aspect of divine love, our modern culture considers sexual love of less spiritual value than divine love. This is exemplified by the virgin-whore dichotomy that polarizes women as either sexual or spiritual. You may have been raised to believe that sexuality is antithetical to spirituality. But imagine how you would perceive yourself and your sexuality if you had learned that it was sacred. If you've felt that you had to make a choice between the two, I want to reassure you that you can deeply appreciate your animal's sexual nature and still be a spiritual woman.

Many religions and spiritual practices promise a profound experience of divine union in which you realize that everything is alive and interconnected and that you are a part of the web of life. But many don't encourage sacred sexuality as the easiest way to achieve this experience of divine union. While it's possible to get to this experience through chanting, fasting, praying, or meditating, the sexual route is more accessible. "In truly good sex, and not just 'a genital sneeze and a release of tension,' you have the experience of being one with all of life. Those are the sorts of experiences that most people would think of as spiritual," says holistic sexuality expert Sheri Winston. The experience of pleasure and ecstasy are inherently sacred. When we are in expanded pleasure states in which we don't know where we end and the universe begins, we are having a direct experience of the divine. That's why many religions are critical of sex; they don't want people to have an unmediated experience of the divine.

PLEASURE PRACTICE
Rock the Camera

It seems that women who struggle with their "weight" dislike two ordinary objects: the mirror and the camera. They tell me all the time, "I don't think I look too bad until I see photos of myself, and then I'm horrified." You may also want to lose weight first, before surrendering your image to the eye of a camera, but as always in the Pleasurable Weight Loss approach, there's a benefit to doing it the other way around. Learning to surrender and relax into your existing beauty catalyzes the relaxation response that triggers weight loss.

So how do you rock it in front of the camera when you are not happy with how you look? Let's begin with a look into a central Hindu concept known as *darshan*. Loosely translated as "vision of the divine," darshan is when a devotee of a Hindu god or goddess goes to a temple or shrine to literally see the deity. The implication in darshan is that you are not looking at a statue or a painting of the god or goddess but rather that you are beholding the real deal, the divine itself. Darshan doesn't stop there, however. Not only are you seeing the divine but also the divine is seeing you!

What if a photograph were an opportunity for darshan? What if when looking at your image, another person could have the experience of seeing the divine feminine in all her glory and at the same time that person could in turn feel seen? That's the power that's available in every photograph. If you think your photos are intended to catalogue only the size of your body, then they won't be very inspiring. Instead, allow your image to be a communication of the rich canvas of the woman you are—alive, full of emotions, and perfectly imperfect.

"But what about my weight?" you may be gasping. "I don't look good like this! Can't you see?" To address this, I invite you to be proud of the journey of your life and to communicate that to the camera. Send a message of radiant beauty by staying grounded in your body as the photos are being taken. This means that you need to stay present in your senses and to the emotions in your heart, instead of attempting to control them or shut them down. Ride the wave and feel everything that comes up. Radiate aliveness and your personal magnetism through your eyes. Aligning with your aliveness and personal magnetism will also heighten your enjoyment of life, which will cause your self-esteem to increase. Loving yourself and your female animal through and through contributes to your happiness and relaxation, establishing the perfect conditions for sustainable and pleasurable weight loss.

YOUR SEXINESS IS A CONTRIBUTION

When you are in direct contact with your pleasure and delight, not only are you more alive, you also have access to the parts of your brain that make you courageous, boost your self-esteem, heighten your creativity, and allow you to function optimally in every realm of life. You are turned on not only in the sexual sense but also as a whole being.

A woman who is deeply connected to her sexuality has a greater capacity to contribute to society. Every woman I've ever met who has been in touch with her pleasure becomes more alive and more connected and inspired to do something magnificent in the world. The natural sexy energy you exude just by being you is sacred. It is a contribution and a gift.

Because of the way the mammalian brain works, we are highly influenced by each other's moods. When someone feels bad, we all feel it. So, when a woman is turned on by life and enjoying the flow of her natural sexy energy, everyone in contact with her feels the positivity. When you are free from sexual shame, other people feel liberated in your presence. It's as if a whole world's weight is lifted, and everyone can enjoy his or her erotic innocence. In this way, your sexual energy can heighten other people's awareness to pleasure and all the healing benefits it bestows.

One of the very nicest things about life is the way we must
regularly stop whatever it is we are doing and devote
our attention to eating.

LUCIANO PAVAROTTI

8 Pleasurable Eating: Nourishing Your Animal

WHEN I TALK about food being pleasurable, I'm not just
referring to your taste buds but also to how food affects your
entire body. When you think about food in this way, you'll
notice more than taste, too. For example, you'll notice whether
specific foods make your female animal feel more energized
and alert or sluggish and dull. Paying attention to additional
sensations like this will guide you to eat the right foods in the
right quantities.

For my client Megan, food had become the object of a love-
hate relationship. On the one hand, food was her friend and a
source of comfort when she found herself alone at the end of a
long day. Yet on the other hand, she cursed it for being the source
of her embarrassing weight gain. Megan worked in the New York
fashion industry where it seemed all the women in her office
aspired to look like runway models. Their idea of a healthy lunch
was a salad and a cigarette.

Megan believed that to lose weight she couldn't eat whatever she wanted. She would have to muster the discipline and

restrict or eliminate foods she loved. By the time she met me, she had gained fifteen pounds, she was anxious and depressed, and she was starting to believe that all foods were her enemy. Like Megan, you might also believe you can't eat what you want if you are ever to lose weight, but that's simply not true. You can eat whatever you want and as much of it as you want. The secret is that it's more important to listen to what your animal wants and follow her guidance than to what your mind thinks you want or need to eat.

Charles Eisenstein, author of *Transformational Weight Loss,* says, "You cannot use your mind to figure out the desires of your body," and I completely agree. Your female animal speaks her own language. Once you start to listen to her and are truly willing to follow her guidance, no matter how long you've struggled with food compulsions, you will find that she knows what to eat, when to eat, and how much to eat. She will communicate to you through sensations and feelings. Your mind's job is to stay present and to be aware of those sensations, bite by bite.

When I struggled with food and weight, I ate until I was full or unpleasantly stuffed. I often didn't stop until I was in a food coma. I wasn't aware at the time that eating this way requires the body to generate more metabolic force for digestion. More oxygen and blood must be sent to the digestive organs, and some of that extra blood flow comes from the head, which is why we feel tired and sluggish after overeating or eating until we feel full. The female animal, however, doesn't want to feel this way. She would much rather be alert and sprightly, with plenty of energy to enjoy the other activities in life.

PLEASURABLE EATING IS NOURISHING

When I lived in India and was still wrestling with a painful relationship to food, I found comfort when I learned about Annapurna, the goddess of food, cooking, and nourishment. As soon as I learned about her existence, I noticed images of her everywhere: tacked on the walls of kitchens and restaurants, or her name sometimes written over the entrance to a kitchen. At that time, food was so fraught with pain and shame for me that learning about a goddess who symbolized the divine aspect of nourishing care was welcome healing.

During that time, I also came across some writings by Amma, an Indian sage who is known as "the hugging Mother." What caught my attention was the blessing she shared for meals: "May I feed myself as if I am feeding the divine within." The message of this blessing was not at all what I thought I was doing. Far from feeding the divine within, I felt like I was feeding a shameful beast living in the darkness of myself. I was so full of self-loathing and shame that every opportunity to eat was another opportunity to hate myself. I shoved food down my throat, fast, furiously, and unconsciously, not in a way at all appropriate for a divine being. Bringing a new consciousness to my eating began when I started to use Amma's blessing before I ate. Today, I continue to use this blessing. This one change led to improvements in my eating experience. The blessing helped me think of food as a source of nourishment instead of shame.

Understanding that we eat for nourishment is another secret of pleasurable weight loss, because what our animals want above all is to be nourished, not overfed. And while fresh, nutrient-dense foods are technically the most nutritious foods, if you bring the intention to be nourished to the table, any meal can become more nourishing. Whether you are at an event where none of the foods your animal prefers to eat are available or you are willfully eating foods that are not so healthy, the food itself is only half of what makes a meal nourishing. The other half comes from the intention you bring to be nourished by the food. This means being present with the food and feeling good about eating it. This practice of awareness will also help you let go of the guilt you feel about eating certain foods; instead, you eat them with pleasure.

PLEASURE BITE

Take part in a time-honored ritual for heightening the pleasure of eating chocolate. First, bring a piece of high-quality chocolate to your nose. Close your eyes and breathe in its aroma. Then, with your eyes closed, place the chocolate in your mouth, and instead of chewing it, let the chocolate melt on your tongue.

DEVELOPING THE RIGHT RELATIONSHIP WITH FOOD

I invite you to have a personal relationship with food, which I've heard described as the most intimate relationship because when food enters your body, it supports all of your cells, tissues, and organs, which in turn support your physical experience, as well as your thoughts, feelings, and emotions. Food's entry into your body should indeed be a sacred experience. So, begin to view food as a valued friend, and let your animal savor the vital experience of eating nourishing foods.

Your mind's role is to be a caretaker who makes sure to locate the highest-quality food for your animal. When you eat food of low nutritional value, you may find that she keeps craving more sustenance. Foods high in nutrients do the reverse; they eliminate cravings. To satisfy her needs, upgrade the quality of your food; whenever possible include organic, locally grown whole foods, which, broadly speaking, are the foods that don't come in packages and are usually found at the perimeter of the grocery store. Fresh fruits and vegetables in season, lean meats and poultry (ideally, free range and/or grass fed), fresh fish, whole grains, beans, nuts and seeds, and fresh dairy are all healthy choices. When you upgrade the quality of your food, weight loss will naturally follow.

One of the ironies of the Western world is that we can be both malnourished and overweight. I was shocked when I first learned this: I thought if someone was overweight (me at the time), she was also overnourished. But it turns out that overeating high-calorie, processed foods can cause us to excrete more nutrients than we take in. You've probably heard the term *empty calories,* which refers to foods primarily made of sugar, refined flour, and low-quality oils, devoid of nutritional value. But it's actually a more sinister dynamic than that. That's why I refer to low-nutrient foods not as empty calories but as "thieving calories," because they steal from your animal's nutrient reserves in order to be digested. When her nutrient resources are low, your animal doesn't have the right hormonal balance to support weight loss, good mood, sleep, sexual health, and overall vitality. You can't feed your body low-quality food and expect her to shine. If you are overweight and malnourished, you can replenish your body with high-nutrient foods. As you start to eat fresher, more vibrant foods, you will immediately notice a difference.

Your animal is not designed to handle "a high-fact diet." She does not need to be force-fed contradictory nutritional information. A ton of information is thrown at us every day about which foods to eat and which to avoid, as well as how much is too much or not enough. When information overload makes you anxious, you are no longer serving the best interests of your animal. That's why I'm simply focusing on quality food, not a detailed prescription. Eat the foods your animal desires, and she will support your weight loss. No matter what the experts are saying, your animal's deeper wisdom, accessed in a state of relaxation, always has the final word.

For example, your animal evolved to be omnivorous long before the politics of veganism or vegetarianism existed. In my experience, it's not only less satisfying and less pleasurable to exclude meat and fish from our diet, it's not the way our bodies are designed to function. For seven years, when I was in my late teens to mid-twenties, I was a vegetarian and I thought I was doing the right thing for my body and Mother Earth. When I first made the shift, I initially felt more energized; this new way of eating was like a detoxification. But over time that energy faded away and I was left struggling with sugar cravings, fatigue, and my weight. Even so, I hung on to the vegetarian dogma: my mind was convinced that I was making the best choice. It wasn't until I was in nutrition school, debating vegetarianism versus omnivorism, that some classmates dared me to experiment with eating meat again. Taking up the challenge, I went to the health food store and bought some high-quality meat. To my great surprise, I perked up. The very next day I woke before my alarm clock and felt more energized than I had in years. That was when I understood my animal's needs weren't "politically correct." I wasn't hearing what she was asking for because I was convinced my mind knew better. But when I gave her what she required—which turned out to be a full range of proteins, carbohydrates, and healthy fats—I was able to feel physically better, and finally shed twenty pounds. If you're a vegan or vegetarian and are still struggling with your weight and food cravings, I encourage you to put your philosophical views aside and—with a pleasure-positive attitude—experiment with eating high-quality animal proteins to see how your body responds.

The act of eating triggers pleasure chemistry: no matter what you eat, as long as you enjoy it, you are going to release endorphins that make you feel good. Remember, every pleasurable experience increases your metabolism. This means that there is a place for dessert and even refined foods. Humans are meant to be omnivores. We are designed to enjoy all types of food, including the sweets and fats that so many of us have been taught to fear and avoid. In fact, the foods that cause the strongest endorphin response typically contain 50 percent fat and 50 percent sugar—ice cream and chocolate fit this category. However, once you incorporate lots of different, healthy food choices into your diet, and put attention on deriving maximum pleasure while you eat, then you'll also find that the healthiest foods can be equally satisfying.

Psychologist Alia Crum created an experiment that confirms what I'm saying. She wanted to know whether the way you think about food changes the body's physiological response. Crum created a milkshake that she divided into two pitchers with different labels. One was labeled a no-fat, no-added-sugar drink with 140 calories per serving. The other was labeled a rich treat with 620 calories per serving. In truth, all the shakes had 300 calories each. Crum found that if people believed they were drinking the rich shake, they were more satisfied and less hungry than when they thought they were drinking the low-cal shake. Her research shows how powerful the mind is; our beliefs strongly influence metabolic response. For pleasurable weight loss, this means that if you think your food is purely functional and low in pleasure, your body will be less satisfied. You'll be hungrier sooner and searching for food again. However, if you believe your food is a pleasurable indulgence, no matter how healthy it is, you'll be completely satisfied.

Food is meant to be nourishing, not a source of shame, stress, or punishment. This is why I want you to enjoy all of your meals. Accept that your body was designed to enjoy fats and sweets and let go of the guilt that is literally toxic for weight loss. What brings you pleasure is never evil when eaten in the right amount, which your animal will determine. The goal of pleasurable weight loss is to create a natural relationship with all types of food so that you recognize what you want to eat in the present moment and food does not become a preoccupation or an afterthought.

PLEASURE PRACTICE
Focus on Foods You Love

Write down all the foods that give you pleasure, even if they are not considered "good" for you. Then create a second list of the foods you find pleasurable that are considered "good" for you. Make the foods on these two lists the basis of your weekly shopping list. Don't waste your money on diet foods you don't like, and don't forbid yourself from eating the foods that bring you pleasure. Just make sure that whatever you eat is what your animal truly wants.

YOUR INNER ECOLOGY AND FEAR OF FOOD

Most women who are struggling with weight are scared of their appetites being too big. They're afraid they want too much and will overeat. Actually, your appetite is commensurate with your metabolism. So if you're truly hungry, you will have the metabolic power to digest and metabolize the food you eat.

Women who take appetite suppressants to dull their hunger are unintentionally suppressing their metabolism at the same time. You can't suppress your appetite and not suppress your metabolism. This approach impedes pleasurable weight loss. That's why if you skip lunch and have a cup of coffee to quiet your appetite instead, you are actually not doing yourself a weight loss favor. So when you feel your appetite come on, instead of allowing that sensation to trigger the fear of overeating, I invite you to reprogram your thinking. This sensation is a positive indicator of your body's metabolism, which you should respond to with respect and attention. It's only when you feel ashamed of your appetite and are not fully present when you eat that you will more likely overeat. When you pay attention to your true appetite, you can eat to your heart's content.

It is fascinating to learn that our fear of food can actually cause us to gain weight, before we even eat it. Let's say that you walk past an ice cream parlor and think, "I love ice cream, and I'd love to eat some right now. But I shouldn't have it because it's fattening." Just this thought, "I want it, but I can't have it," creates stress in the body, which can cause you to gain weight. So without even eating a bite, you can put yourself in a state that prevents you from losing weight.

Don't be afraid that your appetite will lead you to ruin. Your appetite is your personal metaphor for everything in life: your sexual appetite, your appetite for love, and your appetite for freedom. When you embrace your appetite you give yourself the right to want what you want. Make a pact with your animal that you will never starve her again.

Also, you may notice that your appetite changes at different times of the month and the year. This is normal. In the colder seasons, your animal will want to eat more and will favor warmer, heavier foods. In the warmer seasons, you'll be drawn to lighter, raw, and more cooling foods. When you pay attention and stay curious, your animal's cravings will show you when it's time to adjust your food choices.

PLEASURE BITE

At my Pleasure Camps, I teach participants how to awaken their senses of smell, taste, and touch, connecting them to the act of eating by using a blindfold. Experiment with eating your favorite treats or even a whole meal this way. You may be surprised by how much pleasure you receive.

HUNGER IS A SENSATION GAME

I used to be terrified of the sensation of getting really hungry—so I would eat in advance to preempt the feeling. Other women have told me they feel the same way: that the sensation of hunger triggers fear. In Chapter 5 we spoke about sensations, the meanings we give them, and how sensations trigger beliefs. The most common belief triggered by the feeling of hunger is the fear of scarcity, a fear of not having or not being enough. The underlying fear of scarcity could apply to anything—money, love, happiness, all of which can tie into being hungry. If you fear there will not be enough food, you can't relax into your animal's natural appetite because you will be stressed and your body will ward off the potential threat by bulking up. In this case, overeating has nothing to do with food but with a deeper belief about not having or being enough, and overeating needs to be addressed on this level. (If this is your issue, review Chapter 6.)

As the years have gone by, I've noticed that now I can tolerate hunger without triggering a stress response or needing to address it by eating immediately. I don't ignore the hunger; I acknowledge it and tell my animal: "I know you're hungry. I'm not denying you but allowing your appetite to build. Then we will eat." When my hunger crosses a certain threshold, I know I must feed my animal.

My client Dominique went from a size 10 to a size 4 once I taught her to honor her hunger and respect her animal. She was the chief finance officer of a construction company and was frequently the only woman on a job site. The men would drink coffee and eat donuts and not stop for proper meals, and she felt the pressure to do the same. Because of our work together, she learned to tell the men, "This animal's got to eat," as she walked off a site to seek out real food. "When I said it like that, they all respected my choice, and no one gave me a hard time," she reported proudly.

PLEASURABLE EATING PRACTICE 8
Breathe While You Eat

As you eat, breathe consciously through your nose and enjoy your food at a relaxed pace. I can't emphasize enough the power of consciously breathing while you are chewing to completely change your relationship to food. If you've struggled with emotional eating, as I did, then you may feel skeptical about this simple technique, but I assure you it works better than almost anything I've come across.

As you continue to pay attention to breathing deeply and staying present with the experience of eating, you will become more relaxed, and the more relaxed you are, the more sensitized to pleasure you become. At first it may feel odd, like you are trying to rub your belly and pat your head at the same time, but you'll quickly get used to it. The result is that you will become satisfied sooner and will eat less. The reason is that you don't need the food to get you to a relaxed state.

Every few minutes put down your fork, and take a mini breath and relaxation break. Check in with your animal and make sure you are still hungry. Stop chewing, and continue breathing deeply, savoring the smell of the food and allowing yourself to relax into the experience.

Cultivating the practice of conscious breathing can enhance anything you do. For example, breathing consciously while you are being sensual or sexual also opens the gateway to greater heights of pleasure.

A TRUTH ABOUT FOOD CRAVINGS

You think certain foods have power over you, but they don't. The truth is, you are the one with the power. Some people have "trigger foods"—for example, "If I eat a bite of ice cream, I am going to want to eat the whole pint." If it helps you to keep certain foods out of the house, do so, but keep in mind that the ultimate goal is to be connected to what truly nourishes your animal and to trust her to lead you to make good decisions. There was a time I couldn't keep chocolate in my house for even one night without devouring it; now I can have a chocolate bar in my pantry for weeks, as I enjoy it piece by piece.

When you follow the Pleasurable Weight Loss approach, you won't be searching for low-fat or fat-free foods in an effort to slim down. Low-fat eating is nothing more than a fad, which can be debilitating for your health if you fall for it. In typical low-fat or no-fat products, the fat that is removed is then replaced by sugar, making these foods a poor choice for your animal. There's nothing worse for a woman's body than a no-fat diet. If you've been on one, you know how awful you felt: mood swings, irritability, depression, cravings, low energy, dry or oily skin, constipation, poor digestion, and, yes, you guessed it, weight gain—not weight loss. Depriving your animal of fats will not help your metabolism become more efficient, which is the name of the game for plea-surable and sustainable weight loss.

If you find you have strong fat cravings, it is because fat, like sugar, gives us a strong pleasure hit in the form of endorphins. You crave fat because it brings you pleasure. In some instances, I believe that fat cravings are a sensuality craving in disguise, just like Amelia craved chocolate cake, milkshakes, and French fries when she really wanted a sensual physical connection. Your animal might be asking for something luxurious and rich, but not nec-essarily in the form of food. Rubbing a beautifully scented oil on your body—whether you do it yourself, or someone does it for you—can be one of the most pleasurable, relaxing experiences. Perfect times to do this are when you are fresh out of the shower, before you pleasure yourself, at the end of the day before drifting off to sleep, or when you are receiving a professional massage. If women spent more time having oil rubbed on their bodies, there would be fewer women compulsively eating greasy foods like chips and fries because their animal's pleasure quota would be met.

Sometimes a craving for food, especially sugar, is a thirst for water in disguise. The human body is composed of nearly 60 percent water, and our bodies are acutely sensitive to its absence. As you learn to attune to your need for fresh water, you'll know that when you have a food craving, you might want to offer your animal a glass of water before you devour that chocolate bar. I rec-ommend having your own nondisposable water bottle in a style and color you enjoy carrying around. Making hydration a deeply rooted habit is important for a happy animal.

Sugar cravings are not limited to sweets; they can also include baked goods and other wheat-based foods, especially those made with white flour. Switching from white-flour products, like breads and pasta, to whole-grain flour products, or better yet, to whole grains in their whole form, will stabilize your blood sugar levels, which can combat cravings. Some women find that eating gluten-free grain products is best for their animals; no gluten makes them feel lighter and more energetic. Some people veer toward the ancient grains, which are less processed than wheat, such as amaranth, buckwheat, kamut, millet, quinoa, and spelt. Some people do better with little to no grains in their diet; they are not restricting themselves but rather responding to how their animals feel. Experiment with any of these grain alternatives and see what best supports your pleasurable weight loss.

The mind and body need to work together to get past food cravings. For example, a craving for salt can be an indication of a craving for trace minerals that were once found in sea salt. Your animal is not able to say, "I need iodine," so with her cravings, she lets you know that she needs you to eat salt to get the needed iodine. Plain table salt is now devoid of trace minerals, however; so eating salty chips or shaking extra table salt on your food won't fulfill the nutrient craving. What you'll find is you're compelled to eat more of these foods, and the vicious cycle of eating but never being satisfied ensues. Breaking such a cycle requires the partnership of mind and body to help your body get what's needed with educated choices.

HAVE A PLEASURABLE RELATIONSHIP WITH ALCOHOL

Many restrictive diets require you to give up alcohol in order to lose weight. The reason is that wine, beer, and hard liquors are full of sugar, which offers no nutritional value. However, alcohol is an ancient source of pleasure that we know generates the relaxation response. When it adds to your quality of life, it can have a place in your pleasurable weight loss. The secret is to figure out whether you are drinking for true pleasure or counterfeit pleasure.

On the path of pleasurable weight loss, every woman will have a unique relationship with alcohol. Alcohol does not agree with everyone, just as all foods don't agree with everyone. You'll need to pay close attention to how your animal responds while you are drinking and hours later. Some women can happily enjoy a few glasses of wine, while others don't feel well after one drink. Alcohol might give you a headache, interrupt your sleep, or exacerbate menopausal symptoms like hot flashes. If drinking makes your female animal feel bad, then it's not a true pleasure.

Drinking alcohol can be a true pleasure when it complements a meal or when you drink responsibly to enjoy or celebrate an occasion. Contrary to the idea that drinking will cause you to overeat, when you approach alcohol as a true pleasure, the opposite can occur. Pleasure expert and wine connoisseur Tonya Leigh told me, "I use alcohol as a way to bring out more pleasure from my food. When you pair beautiful wines with beautiful foods, you get an even more pleasurable experience. When I have a glass of wine with dinner, I end up eating less because my senses are more engaged. I'm getting more pleasure from my food as the wine brings out more of the flavors, and as a result I'm satisfied sooner."

If you're waking up with a hangover or if you find you overeat when you drink, those are signs that your relationship with alcohol is not serving your animal and needs to change. While drinking alcohol can be relaxing, make sure that when you do, your animal's vitality is heightened rather than dulled. If your intention with alcohol is to feel less rather than feel more, then you are using alcohol as a counterfeit pleasure. Drinking in excess to avoid difficult issues that are also holding you back from losing weight won't give you what you want. Real solutions will only come through genuine healing.

THE HEALING POWERS OF FOOD AND THE SIX TASTES

The most dangerous outcome of the punishing approach to weight loss is that food becomes your enemy. Punishing diets are inflexible, restrict specific food groups, reduce food to numbers, and overlook what some Eastern traditions already know: that food is medicine. Certain foods are good for the liver, others benefit the lungs, and still others help digestion. When you can start to get to know the ways food helps you, instead of focusing only on the ways food makes you fat, then a whole new world will open up where food can be your healing ally. One of the defining features of the pleasurable approach to weight loss is a sensitivity to what your body experiences, which then guides your food choices.

In contrast, the pleasurable approach to weight loss is completely flexible. We evolved to be omnivores and can take pleasure in all types of healthy foods. Colorful fruits and vegetables are high in antioxidants that keep you healthy. Foods high in both animal and vegetable proteins provide lots of energy and keep your brain focused. Healthy fats keep you feeling satisfied, as well as making your hair silky and shiny and your skin supple. They also support memory and a healthy libido, and make sex juicier. In my opinion, it is less pleasurable to exclude meat, poultry, or dairy from our diets because these are the foods that make us feel full and support a healthy body. I also think it's harder to lose weight sustainably if you are a vegetarian or a vegan because it's more difficult to get the protein and saturated fat that you need to support your animal's well-being.

One way to explore the healing properties of food is through different tastes.

When I was struggling with food and weight, I classified food in black and white categories: fattening or nonfattening, good or bad. My understanding ended there, and metrics never helped me because I was playing the weight loss game in my head. Once I connected with food directly through my senses and paid careful attention to how it made me feel, I was able to finally lose weight and keep it off.

Ayurveda, the traditional healing system from India, categorizes food into six tastes, each of which can elicit a specific bodily response. It defines a balanced meal as one that incorporates each of them. The six tastes are *sweet* (fruit, grains, honey, sugar), *sour* (yogurt, lemons, vinegar), *salty* (olives, soy sauce, sea salt), *pungent* (ginger, wasabi, spicy foods, onions, radishes), *bitter* (dark green leafy vegetables and eggplant), and *astringent* (lentils, most beans, pomegranate, aloe vera juice).

Depending on your body's constitution, Ayurveda recommends emphasizing certain tastes more than others. For example, if you are struggling with weight or frequently suffer from heavy, depressive moods, emphasize the pungent, bitter, and astringent tastes. Make sure those three flavors are featured in the foods you eat on a regular basis. These are the three least popular of the common tastes and are not typically found in modern convenience foods, so they are the easiest to miss.

I find that using the taste of foods as a guide, rather than a numerical measurement, gets me out of my head and into my body because the only way to discern taste is to be present to the senses.

PLEASURE PRACTICE
Explore the Six Tastes

Exploring food through taste is so much more fun than analyzing meals for calorie content. What tastes do you gravitate toward? What tastes do you avoid? Experiment with the sweet, sour, salty, pungent, bitter, and astringent flavors in new ways. Using condiments such as lemon, hot sauce, sauerkraut, or seaweed flakes is an easy way to incorporate these six flavors into otherwise simple meals. Ideally, include all six flavors throughout the course of a day. In the next chapter, where I share dozens of recipes, note the ingredients that match each of the six tastes. Try keeping a food journal of flavors where you list which tastes were present in the day's meals.

PLEASURABLE EATING PRACTICE 9
Eating to the Point of Energy

Since we are not going to be measuring our food or counting points or calories with the Pleasurable Weight Loss approach, you're going to check in with your animal to know how much to eat and when to stop. Are you familiar with the recommendation to eat until you are 80 percent full? Although this sounds sensible, I find this advice useless because how on earth can we tell when we've reached that magic 80 perecent? My stomach doesn't have a meter on it, and neither does yours.

What I discovered instead is that the secret is "to eat to the point of energy." In *The Slow Down Diet,* Marc David describes this as a strategic point in the meal, when you are able to walk away from your plate with more energy, or life force, than when you sat down to eat. Identifying this point of energy takes some experimentation, but when you discover it, you'll have unlocked the power of this practice, which is crucial for easy and natural weight loss.

The way this technique works is to pay close attention to your energy level before you eat and as you eat. You'll find that before you eat, your energy is low. That's your body's way of indicating that food is needed. Then, as you eat, your energy will increase, especially when you incorporate all of the Pleasurable Eating Practices. You will feel more alert, less tired, and more energized. When you've had enough to eat, your energy will start to go down. The trick is to stop eating just at the point when you first feel your energy dip. When you've gone even one bite past that point of energy, you'll start to feel heavier and fatigued; that's the indication that it's time to stop. Practice this technique, and you'll soon complete your meals still feeling energetic. You'll feel ready to take on the world, instead of lethargic and ready to go to bed.

To help you recognize this point of energy, as you eat, bite by bite, check in with your animal. See how she is feeling. The more you attend to your animal's sensations, the easier it will be to recognize this sweet spot. Remember, you're not meant to think about whether you are energized but to feel it. Listen to what your animal is telling you. Allow for trial and error as you start to eat intuitively. It's not about getting it right the first time but about experimenting, listening, and beginning to trust.

At first, eating to the point of energy is going to feel much different than you're accustomed to feeling at the end of a meal. You may still feel slightly hungry, especially if you're used to eating yourself into a food coma. You may see that you're leaving uneaten food on the plate. But as you practice, you'll find that eating to the point of energy is a comfortable and pleasurable experience.

This technique, along with the others I share throughout the book, is exactly what pleasurable eating is all about: eating with presence and in partnership with your animal. You're now ready to bring all the practices into play at your meals as you eat to the point of energy:

- Check in with your animal
- Enhance your eating environment
- Relax before you eat
- Smell the food
- Seek pleasure in every bite
- Master the art of chewing
- Eat slowly and sensually
- Breathe while you eat

Cook like your life depends on it, because it does.

JOSHUA ROSENTHAL

9 The Art of Pleasurable Cooking

ONCE FOOD HAS CEASED to be the enemy, you can relax and have fun in the kitchen. Our next step on the path of pleasurable weight loss is pleasurable cooking. You might be thinking, "Who is she kidding? Cooking is not pleasurable." For any busy woman, cooking can easily become another chore on the never-ending to-do list. But it doesn't have to be that way. Cooking is a ripe area to learn to enjoy. It can also make the difference between eating high-quality meals cooked to your animal's preferences and low-quality take-out meals. By applying pleasure principles to cooking, you can have a completely new relationship with it, where it becomes a source of sensual pleasure, nourishment, and feminine pride.

Self-love expert and master chef Michel Madie recommends thinking of cooking as an inexpensive and fun art form, accessible to everyone. Although the average woman will never need to paint, dance, or write poetry, cooking is a need. "Enter the kitchen as if you are going to a dance class, and imagine you are dancing as you swivel from your spice cabinets, to your fridge, to your chopping board," says Michel.

Learning to cook is like learning to play an instrument, but easier. It can take time to learn a new song, but once you can play it and have your groove on, you'll know it forever. Knowing that you're self-sufficient in the kitchen and that you can feed yourself and others builds self-confidence. Creating a beautiful, delicious meal will give you a sense of grounded self-worth. As Julia Child says, in cooking you've got to have a what-the-hell attitude. Let your cooking be an act of improvisation and inspiration.

It's time to bring all your creative feminine powers into the kitchen. When you enter the kitchen, imagine that you are an alchemist making magic out of everyday ingredients. Even if you feel like you can't cook to save your life, it is in your DNA to know how to prepare food. Tens of thousands of generations of women have been cooking, so even if your mother didn't have an appreciation for this skill, you still have an intuitive knack for it. And you can still learn to love it.

Cooking is an opportunity to bond with your animal in a deeply primal way. Even if you are not romancing anyone else, you are always romancing her. You are important enough to cook for. Also, our busy lives don't lend themselves to putting our hands into the earth on a regular basis, so food preparation is a wonderful way to connect with the earth. When you are using fresh, wholesome ingredients, you can feel their life energy moving through your hands. I feel very connected with my primal nature when I have a good sharp knife in my hand and I am cutting into flesh, be it fruit, vegetable, or animal.

Cooking allows us to be in the present moment and to slow down. Let yourself bathe in the sensuality of the kitchen as you explore color, texture, taste, and aroma. It is a fun, joyful, and playful adventure of the senses. "Cooking causes us to become more sensual creatures," says Pamela Morgan, a culinary expert who teaches men and women how to use food to generate romance. Cooking is an opportunity to get into the kitchen with friends, lovers, and family. Pamela says, "Make it playful. Have a good time doing some cutting and chopping together. It will take your relationships to a whole different level."

Cooking dinner is the most challenging meal for women because they're already tired and hungry. If you are so hungry that you are irritable and don't have the patience to cook, that can be a sign that you have not eaten enough during the day. Next time, have a bigger lunch or a snack later in the day before dinner. Alexandra Jamieson, chef and author of *Women, Food, and Desire,* says, "If you get home and you are already hungry, it's okay to eat a snack of fruit or nuts or to have a cup of tea while you cook." Let's also clarify that food does not have to be gourmet to be pleasurable; simple meals have a delightful pleasure of their own. Alexandra Jamieson says, "Keep it simple. Simplicity equals pleasure. Then move on to more complicated things once you've mastered the simplest meals."

When you hear "pleasurable cooking," you might think that it will be time consuming. Women often say that the reason they don't cook is they don't have enough time, but cooking can be more efficient than eating out. What's more, some of the most pleasurable dishes require the simplest cooking. A meal can be as simple as three or four quality ingredients put together with a bit of care and attention—and that can take five minutes. Once you are proficient in the kitchen, cooking doesn't have to be time consuming, and the time you do spend cooking feels creative and nourishing. Having control over the ingredients that go into your meals will also make you healthier. For example, you decide how much and what kind of oil you'll use and exactly how spicy you want something.

Learning by trial and error is the best and the oldest way to learn how to cook. I still make mistakes—and with a name like la Flamme (which means "the flame"), you can be sure I burn my food from time to time! Start learning some basic techniques using the recipes in this chapter, and build on that. Eventually, you'll have a great repertoire.

CREATING A KITCHEN SANCTUARY

You want to make sure you feel comfortable and grounded while you cook, so create an atmosphere you feel at ease in. Make your kitchen a sanctuary. Make it a haven of healing and creativity that you enjoy spending time in so that you look forward to using it.

Let your kitchen have style and not just be purely functional. Paint the cabinets a color you love. Hang art on the wall. Have a vase with fresh flowers on your table. Bring in plants or pots of fresh herbs so that your kitchen feels alive. I like the visual of storing dry ingredients in glass jars instead of plastic packaging. I love to play music and sing along while I cook, so I have an iPod dock. Just as they put altars in the kitchen in India to honor the sacredness of food, create your own kitchen altar with natural objects, candles, incense, or images that inspire you. Use this sacred space to focus your intention on nourishing your animal before you start cooking or eating.

I live in New York City where kitchens are usually small, and space is always a premium. I've learned that when I de-clutter my kitchen so that every drawer and cabinet is a pleasure to behold, I am more comfortable cooking. Alexandra Jamieson shares these three questions to help you know what to keep and what to toss when you are de-cluttering your kitchen: "Do I like this? Do I use it? Is it necessary?" The minimum you'll need is a good sharp knife, a cutting board, and a bowl. The most useful tool in the kitchen is your hands, and those come with you wherever you go. Have some large bowls so you can get your hands involved and you can make big batches of things. Bowls made of natural materials like bamboo and wood are extra pleasurable. Invest in one good knife and keep it sharp so it will cut and chop quickly and easily. Once you are organized and feel more connected to your tools, the kitchen will feel like a place you want to be.

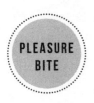

PLEASURE BITE

Explore a local farmer's market. Unlike a supermarket where most fruits and vegetables are available throughout the year, shopping at the farmer's market will teach you to appreciate which fresh vegetables and fruits are in season in your local ecology. For extra pleasure, flirt with the farmers as you create a personal connection with the men and women who grow your food.

CREATING A PLEASURABLE PANTRY

The ritual of cooking begins with its preparation, and that means having the right ingredients on hand. Become familiar with spices and exotic condiments to add flavor to all types of healthy dishes. Alexandra Jamieson suggests, "If someone is new to cooking, choose one recipe a week that is in the flavor profile that you like (Thai, Indian, Italian.) Each recipe will call for a new spice or herb. As you start exploring slowly and with attention, you'll start expanding the spices you have in your kitchen. You don't need to do everything at once. It can be a gentle exploration, bit by bit, of what you like."

I recommend that you find a grocery store that you feel really great about, so that you can get pleasure out of shopping. As Alexandra Jamieson says, "Go to the place you are most excited to go. Give yourself the pleasure of going somewhere that has something juicy for you. If you like talking to the farmer at the farmer's market, go there. Or maybe it's a place where they put attention to stacking the produce in a beautiful way. Whichever place lights you up, go there." If you have a health food store nearby, that's where I recommend you go. Let pleasure be your guide every step of the way, including picking out your food. When you are choosing fresh produce, pick out what looks and smells best to you.

When I was making the transition into healthy eating, I embraced the fairly foolproof, back-to-basics cooking strategy of preparing plain foods like steamed vegetables and whole grains complemented by condiments. Keeping plenty of condiments handy allows you to add whatever flavors you desire to your food, making even the plainest meals taste sumptuous. Avoid artificial sweeteners (Splenda and aspartame) and white sugar; sweeten your foods instead with nutrient-dense maple syrup, brown rice syrup, or raw honey. Stevia is also a great option. And don't be scared of eating or cooking with healthy fats, including full-fat dairy products, coconut oil, extra-virgin olive oil, and sesame oil.

The following list contains great staples for any pantry and includes all of the dry ingredients for the recipes in this chapter:

- Agave nectar
- Alfalfa sprouts
- All-purpose gluten-free flour
- Almond butter
- Almond flour
- Almond milk
- Almond oil
- Almonds
- Amaranth
- Apple cider vinegar

- Apple juice
- Applesauce
- Arame seaweed
- Avocado oil
- Baking powder
- Baking soda
- Balsamic vinegar
- Barley
- Basil
- Bay leaf
- Black beans
- Black pepper
- Bragg's amino acids
- Breadcrumbs
- Brown basmati rice
- Brown rice
- Brown rice flour
- Brown rice syrup
- Cacao powder
- Capers
- Caraway seeds
- Cashew butter
- Cashews
- Cayenne pepper
- Chia seeds
- Chili powder
- Cilantro
- Cinnamon
- Coconut flakes
- Coconut flour
- Coconut manna
- Coconut milk
- Coconut oil
- Coconut water
- Cornmeal
- Corn tortillas
- Cumin
- Curry powder
- Dill
- Dried cherries
- Dry green lentils
- Edible flowers
- Extra-virgin olive oil
- Flaxseed oil
- Flaxseeds
- Garbanzo beans
- Garlic
- Garlic powder
- Ginger
- Gluten-free flatbread (such as corn tortillas)
- Gomasio (a sesame seed and sea salt condiment found in health food stores)
- Grapeseed oil
- Ground ginger
- Hemp seed oil
- Hemp seeds
- Honey
- Hot sauce
- Kalamata olives
- Kumquats
- Lemon juice
- Lentils
- Maca powder
- Maple syrup
- Millet
- Nori seaweed sheets
- Nutmeg
- Nutritional yeast
- Oat flour
- Oats
- Paprika
- Parmesan cheese
- Parsley
- Peanut butter

- Peanut oil
- Peanuts
- Pecans
- Polenta (corn meal)
- Pumpkin puree
- Pumpkin seeds
- Quinoa
- Quinoa pasta
- Raisins
- Raw pumpkin seeds
- Raw sunflower seeds
- Red curry paste
- Rice vermicelli noodles
- Rice vinegar
- Rosemary
- Sea salt
- Seaweed sprinkles or flakes
- Sesame oil
- Sesame seeds
- Shredded unsweetened coconut
- Spirulina
- Sun-dried tomatoes
- Sunflower seeds
- Sunflower sprouts
- Sushi rice
- Tahini paste
- Tamari soy sauce
- Tapioca starch
- Thyme
- Tomato purée
- Tomato sauce
- Tuna, packed in olive oil
- Turmeric
- Umeboshi vinegar
- Unsweetened baking chocolate
- Vanilla extract
- Walnuts
- White pepper
- White vinegar
- Whole wheat pasta
- Wild rice
- Xanthan gum powder
- Zahatar (found in Middle Eastern stores)

PLEASURE PRACTICE
The Ritual of Tea

If you are looking to break ingrained eating patterns or compulsions, you can create new rituals. The ritual of making tea can become a basis for new rituals you create with other foods. I recommend that you stock up on a collection of herbal teas and invest in an attractive teapot. I have an orb-shaped, brushed-metal teapot that I found in a store in Amsterdam that I have been in love with for years. I take deep pleasure in brewing myself a cup of tea in my beautiful teapot and then drinking it out of a cup I love, too.

PLEASURABLE EATING PRACTICE 10
Offering Gratitude to Complete the Meal

Conclude every meal with gratitude. Just as you began the meal in an intentional way by connecting with the wise, feminine life force of your animal, intentionally end the meal with a ritual offering of thanks. This is a way to bring closure to your meal, so that you recognize the feeling of completion.

Thank the earth for the nourishing food she provided; thank the people whose effort went into preparing it, growing it, and bringing it to you; thank your animal for digesting the food; and your mind for making choices that support her. Give thanks in a way that is meaningful to you.

Here's an example of a gratitude prayer inspired by spiritual teacher Javier Regueiro:

Thank you, Mother. Thank you, Father.

Thank you for all the blessings we have received today.

Thank you for all the blessings we receive every day, in every moment of our lives.

Thank you for the air we breathe.

Thank you for the food of every day.

Thank you for the opportunity to eat this meal and spend my life with my female animal.

Thank you to all the plants and animals that nourish us not only in body but also in spirit.

Thank you for the sun, the moon, and the stars, the waters of our rivers, and oceans, snow, and rains.

Thank you for the love, support, friendship, and kindness of family, loved ones, friends, and strangers, close and far away, but always in our hearts.

Thank you, sacred pleasure, for the healing we receive through you and for supporting us to remember our own true divine loving nature.

Thank you, Pacha Mama, Mother Earth.

Thank you for bringing us here and welcoming us.

Thank for taking such good care of us.

And thank you for guiding us on for the rest of our journey on this planet.

PLEASURE BITE

Write down the ten Pleasurable Eating Practices on a beautiful piece of paper, and hang it on your refrigerator or kitchen wall. This will gently remind you of the steps you need to take as you eat.

TEN QUICK STEPS TO A PLEASURABLE SALAD

Salad is the classic diet food that is often perceived as a punishment for being overweight. But this does not have to be the case. Salads can be extremely satisfying. Not only can you eat as much salad as your animal wants but also, with a little creativity, you'll find salads can be an immense source of sensual pleasure. A truly enjoyable salad includes a variety of colors, flavors, aromas, and textures. Made with fresh vegetables, a good salad is vibrant, not limp and lifeless. It's a visual wonder and a gustatory adventure that features a dressing that unifies all the ingredients with an extra sparkle of flavor.

The foundation of a salad is raw greens, one of the healthiest food sources on the planet. Beyond that, you can take it in any direction you want. Use the pleasurable salad guide that follows to inspire you to invent new creations daily in your kitchen. Once you associate salad with pleasure, and not with punishment, you will be eating salad more often with more delight. Invest in a salad bowl and servers that appeal to you, so the whole experience will be a feast of the senses.

1. **Choose greens that you like, and make your life easier by purchasing prewashed greens when you can.** A great salad can start with a favorite green or a medley of favorites—arugula, baby spinach, kale, romaine, and mixed spring greens among them.

2. **Include seeds.** Seeds add extra crunch and flavor, plus protein. Try some of these: black sesame seeds, chia seeds, ground flaxseeds, hemp seeds, pumpkin seeds, sunflower seeds, and white sesame seeds.

3. **Add more protein.** Animal and plant proteins make salads more filling and add vital nutrients that support weight loss. Choose among the following cooked options:

- Beans
- Beef
- Cheese
- Chicken
- Fish
- Lamb
- Quinoa
- Shellfish
- Tempeh
- Tofu
- Turkey

4. **Include sweet vegetables.** Many vegetables are deliciously sweet when you eat them raw. Grate them or slice them into small pieces. They add fabulous color, too. Experiment with beets, carrots, corn (raw or cooked, and cut directly off the cob when available), and fresh peas.

5. **Include fruits.** Don't worry about rules that say we shouldn't eat fruits and vegetables together. Fruits are a great complement to salad greens. Here are some ideas for you to try:
   - Apple, chopped or grated
   - Grapes, halved, seeds removed
   - Papaya slices
   - Mandarin orange sections
   - Tomatoes
   - Dried cherries
   - Pear, chopped or grated
   - Mango slices
   - Blood orange sections
   - Grapefruit sections, pits removed
   - Dried cranberries
   - Raisins

6. **Be daring and add some spicy and pungent flavors.** A little bit of heat in your salad can bring it to a whole new level. Some of these vegetables also have properties that dissolve fat, mucus, and cholesterol, so you derive therapeutic benefits, as well as flavor. If you are not accustomed to these flavors, start by adding a little until you become accustomed to them: daikon radish, grated or sliced; garlic, very finely grated or minced; green onions; mustard greens; red onion; and red radish.

7. **Choose an oil for the base of your salad dressing.** A cold-pressed oil that was created using minimal heat and no chemicals retains the highest amount of nutrients and will be more flavorful. Choose one of the following: almond oil,

avocado oil, extra-virgin olive oil, flaxseed oil, grapeseed oil, hemp seed oil, peanut oil, or walnut oil.

8. **Include tart and tangy flavors in your dressing.** If you pay close attention to your appetite, you may notice that you crave a sour taste. Rather than fulfill it with sea salt and vinegar chips, add tartness to your salads. Combine any of the following ingredients with extra-virgin olive oil to enjoy some tantalizing tang: fresh lemon juice, fresh lime juice, and all types of vinegar, especially balsamic vinegar, apple cider vinegar, and umeboshi vinegar.

9. **Include sweet flavors in your dressing.** Greens often taste bitter, and if you are used to more processed foods, some of the flavors of raw vegetables might be unfamiliar. A wonderful trick that I use with my own salads is to add some sweetness to the dressing. Mix a little bit of a natural sweetener in with the oil and vinegar to make a dressing that laces the salad with a hint of sweetness and that rounds out all the other flavors, too. Try some of these: agave syrup, maple syrup, raw honey, and stevia.

10. **Add edible flower blossoms.** Flowers add a new dimension of beauty, making the simplest dish gourmet. You can grow nasturtiums in your window to add to your salads, buy edible flowers at the health food store, or learn which flowering plants in your natural environment are edible so that you can harvest them. I once picked pink cherry blossoms right from my neighbor's tree and put them in my salad. Try some of these: day lily, lavender, nasturtiums, pansy, squash blossoms, and zucchini blossoms.

A WEEK OF PLEASURABLE EATING: THE RECIPES

Here are my favorite recipes, which will cover three meals a day for one full week—plus snacks and desserts. Ideally, lunch should be the biggest meal of your day because your metabolic power is most efficient when the sun is high in the sky. However, what's most important is that you maintain a regular and reliable eating rhythm and that you don't skip meals. The more consistent your eating pattern is, the more regular and reliable your fat-burning capability will be.

After you prepare your meals, use the Pleasurable Eating Practices. Create a pleasurable eating environment by sitting at a table, not on the couch. Clear the table of clutter. Use pretty plates and cloth napkins. Maybe light a candle or two. Turn off the TV. Turn off your phone. Step away from the computer screen. Savor and relish every bite of your food.

BREAKFAST

WORTH-THE-WAIT MUESLI

This delicious breakfast needs to be made the night before, but it's worth it!
Serves 2

Ingredients
- 1 c. oats
- ¼ c. raisins
- ¼ c. sliced almonds
- ¼ c. sunflower seeds
- ⅛ c. shredded unsweetened coconut
- ½ tsp. cinnamon
- ¼ tsp. nutmeg
- ¼ tsp. sea salt
- 1 can coconut milk
- ½ apple, grated
- 1 tbsp. chia seeds
- fresh berries
- maple syrup

Instructions
In a medium-sized bowl, combine oats, raisins, almonds, sunflower seeds, shredded coconut, cinnamon, nutmeg, and

sea salt. Stir in coconut milk, apple, and chia seeds. Refrigerate overnight. In the morning, give the muesli a good stir. Spoon out a one-cup serving of the mixture into a separate bowl. Top with fresh berries and a drizzle of maple syrup.

STONE FRUIT MILLET PORRIDGE

This porridge provides a hearty flavor sensation that's a grounding way to start the day.

Serves 2

Ingredients

- 1 c. millet
- 1½ c. apple juice
- 1½ c. water
- ¼ tsp. cinnamon
- pinch of sea salt
- 1 tbsp. coconut oil
- ¼ c. almonds
- ¼ c. walnuts
- 2 plums or other stone fruit, thinly sliced
- 2 tbsp. honey
- 1 tsp. shredded coconut

Instructions

Place millet, apple juice, and water in a medium pot, and bring to a boil. Add cinnamon and pinch of sea salt, and cover, bringing heat to medium low. Cook until liquid is absorbed—about a half-hour.

Meanwhile, in a separate pan, heat coconut oil at medium high. When oil is hot, add almonds and walnuts, and sauté until they begin to brown. Add plums and 1 tbsp. honey, turning heat to low. Stirring occasionally, cook until plums are soft and can be cut with the side of a spoon. Set aside.

When millet is cooked through, uncover and stir in plum mixture. Add 1 tsp. shredded coconut and 1 tbsp. honey, and serve.

Optional creamy toppings such as Greek yogurt or almond milk make delicious final touches.

SAUSAGE WITH STEAMED MUSTARD GREENS AND SWEET POTATO HASH

Be curious, and experiment with eating more protein in a savory dish for breakfast. See how your body responds.

Serves 2

Ingredients

- 2 tbsp. olive oil
- 2 sweet potatoes, chopped into small cubes
- 2 cloves garlic, minced
- 1 onion, finely chopped
- ½ tsp. dried rosemary or 1 tsp. chopped fresh rosemary when available
- 2 sweet Italian sausages (pork or chicken), sliced into ¼-inch rounds
- ½ bunch mustard greens, coarsely chopped
- 1 tsp. balsamic vinegar
- sea salt and pepper to taste

Instructions

In a large pan, heat 1 tbsp. olive oil at medium heat. Add garlic and rosemary and sauté until aromatic. Then add the onion and a pinch of sea salt, and sauté until the onion becomes translucent. Stir in sweet potatoes and sausage, and add 1 tbsp. olive oil. Season with sea salt. Turn heat to medium low and cover pan for 5 minutes to allow sweet potatoes to cook through. If the mixture sticks to the bottom of the pan, drizzle a little bit of water in to add moisture. Stir occasionally and cook until potatoes and onions begin to lightly brown.

Meanwhile, steam mustard greens in a separate pot and set aside. Dress with balsamic vinegar, sea salt, and pepper. Serve with sausages and sweet potato hash.

EGG IN A NEST
Serves 1

Ingredients

1 piece gluten-free or ancient-grains bread
  butter or non-dairy butter spread
1 egg
  salt and pepper to taste
  pinch of paprika
  pinch of cinnamon
¼ cup alfalfa sprouts
1 tsp. sunflower seeds
1 tsp. olive oil
1 lemon wedge
1 tsp. maple syrup

Instructions

Using the rim of a small drinking glass, press a hole in the center of the bread.

Heat a small pat of butter or non-dairy spread in a medium pan until melted. Place bread in pan and crack egg into hole. Sprinkle with salt, pepper, paprika, and cinnamon, and cook on medium heat for about 4 minutes. Flip egg and bread and cook another 4 minutes, sprinkling with additional salt, pepper, paprika, and cinnamon.

To serve, place bread and egg on a plate and top with sprouts, sunflower seeds, or maple syrup. If you prefer a savory dish, drizzle with olive oil and juice from a lemon wedge, and sprinkle with salt.

ZUCCHINI AND CORN TEA BREAD
WITH QUICK PRESERVES

Treat yourself like a queen by starting your day with this breakfast.
Makes 1 loaf, approximately 8 servings

Ingredients

Tea Bread

    1 c. grated zucchini (from about 1 medium zucchini)

    1 c. all-purpose gluten-free flour

    ½ c. cornmeal flour

    2 tsp. baking powder

    ½ tsp. baking soda

    ¾ tsp. xanthan gum powder

    ½ tsp. sea salt

    2 tsp. cinnamon

    ½ c. maple syrup

    ⅓ c. coconut oil, melted

    2 eggs

    ¼ c. unsweetened coconut milk

    1 tsp. fresh lemon juice

    1 tbsp. vanilla extract

Quick Preserves

    1 navel orange, washed, ends trimmed, very finely chopped

    2 tsp. water

    ¼ c. maple syrup

       pinch of turmeric

       pinch of cinnamon

Instructions

Preheat oven to 350 degrees. Grease a standard 9-inch loaf pan
with coconut oil and set aside.

Place the grated zucchini onto paper towels and gently squeeze
out any moisture. Fluff the zucchini with a fork and set aside.

Combine both flours, baking powder, baking soda, xanthan
gum powder, sea salt, and cinnamon in a medium bowl, and
whisk to blend. In another large bowl, add the maple syrup,

coconut oil, eggs, coconut milk, lemon juice, and vanilla. Whisk thoroughly until smooth. Add the dry ingredients to the wet, and beat until combined. Fold in the grated zucchini, reserving a little to sprinkle over the top of the loaf.

Pour batter into loaf pan, sprinkle reserved zucchini on top, and bake for 35 to 40 minutes or until a toothpick inserted in the center of the loaf comes out clean. Cool for 5 minutes in the pan after baking, and then carefully turn out to cool the loaf completely on a rack.

While loaf bakes, you can make the quick preserves. Combine chopped orange, water, and maple syrup in a small pot at medium-high heat. Bring to boil, and stir in turmeric and cinnamon. Let boil for 15 minutes, stirring frequently, until mixture becomes thick. Place mixture in a sterilized jar, close lid tightly, and let cool. Refrigerate to store.

TOMATO AVOCADO TOAST
Avocados are packed with healthy fats and make for a new twist on a traditional breakfast.

Serves 1

Ingredients
- 1 clove garlic, halved width-wise
- 2 slices gluten-free or ancient-grains bread, toasted
- 1 tomato, halved
- ½ avocado, sliced into small cubes
  olive oil
  sea salt and pepper to taste

Instructions
With cut-side down, rub garlic clove onto the top of each piece of toast. Discard garlic. With cut-side down, rub tomato onto toast, squeezing out seeds and juices so top of toast will soften. Pull apart leftover tomato meat and skins with hands, place in a bowl with cubed avocados, and drizzle with olive oil. Add sea salt and pepper to taste, and divide tomato-avocado mixture between each piece of toast, pouring on top. Serve.

OMELET WITH FRESH HERBS

This omelet features radishes, which are distinctly pungent and have fat-dissolving properties. Expand your palate and give them a try.

Serves 1

Ingredients

- 2 eggs
- 1 tbsp. water
  - sea salt and pepper to taste
- ¼ c. fresh basil, chopped
- ¼ c. fresh parsley, chopped
- ⅛ c. fresh cilantro, chopped
- ⅛ c. fresh dill, chopped
- 4 radishes, coarsely chopped
  - juice of ½ lemon
  - sea salt
- 1 tbsp. olive oil

Instructions

Beat eggs together in a small bowl, adding 1 tbsp. water for fluffiness, and sea salt and pepper to taste. In a separate bowl, combine basil, parsley, cilantro, dill, and radishes. Toss in lemon juice and sea salt to taste. Set aside.

In a small- or medium-sized frying pan, heat olive oil at medium heat. When oil is hot, pour egg mixture into pan. Turn heat to medium low. As eggs start to become opaque, use a spatula to keep them from sticking to bottom of pan. When eggs reach desired consistency, spoon herb mixture on top of one side of eggs and fold other half of eggs on top. Transfer to plate and serve.

LUNCH

CASHEW NUT CREAM CONDIMENT

This recipe is delicious spread on bread or crackers. You'll also find it listed in several of the other recipes. You can make this in advance and keep in the refrigerator.

Ingredients

> 1 c. raw cashews
> water
> juice from ½ lemon
> sea salt to taste

Instructions

Soak cashews overnight in water. Next day, drain, rinse, and place in a blender. Add water slowly and blend until reaching desired consistency. Add lemon juice and sea salt. Spoon into a glass jar and refrigerate.

BLACK BEAN AND VEGGIE TACOS WITH FRESH RED SALAD AND CASHEW CREAM

I love eating with my hands, especially foods with a distinct texture, like these colorful tacos.

Serves 2

Ingredients

Beans

> 1 tbsp. grapeseed oil
> 2 cloves garlic, minced
> 1 onion, finely chopped
> ½ tsp. cumin
> 1 can black beans, rinsed thoroughly
> sea salt to taste

Veggies
- 1 tbsp. grapeseed oil
- 2 bell peppers (desired colors), thinly sliced
- 1 onion, thinly sliced
- 1 cup Brussels sprouts, trimmed and chopped into quarters
- sea salt to taste

Fresh Red Salad
- 1½ c. grape tomatoes, halved
- 5 radishes, thinly sliced
- ¼ c. fresh cilantro, chopped
- juice from ½ lime
- sea salt to taste

- 4 corn tortillas, heated in pan until soft
- cashew cream (see recipe)

Instructions

For beans
In a pan, heat oil at medium high. Toss in garlic and onions, turning heat to medium, and sauté until onions become transparent. Stir in cumin, and continue to sauté until mix becomes fragrant. Add beans and sea salt to taste. Reduce heat to low, and let beans simmer until other items are done.

For veggies
Meanwhile, heat oil in a large pan at medium-high heat. Toss in all veggies with sea salt, cover, and reduce heat to medium low. Uncover, and stir veggies occasionally until slightly softened and cooked through, about 5 to 10 minutes. Remove from heat.

For salad
Combine all ingredients in a bowl.

To serve, place 2 tortillas on each plate and add beans, veggies, and salad, drizzling cashew cream on top.

LENTIL SALAD WITH ROASTED SUNCHOKES AND SPINACH DOLMAS

A new take on a traditional Greek staple.

Serves 4

Ingredients

Lentil Salad

1	cup dry green lentils
½	red bell pepper, finely chopped
½	yellow bell pepper, finely chopped
1	small yellow onion, finely chopped
2	garlic cloves, minced
1	bay leaf
1	tbsp. olive oil
5	c. water
1	tsp. sea salt
	juice from ½ lemon
1	bunch parsley, finely chopped

Sunchokes

5	sunchokes (Jerusalem artichokes), sliced into ½-inch pieces
1	tsp. olive oil
¼	tsp. sea salt

Spinach Dolmas

½	c. brown rice
2	tbsp. olive oil
½	yellow onion, finely chopped
2	cloves garlic, minced
½	bunch parsley, chopped
2	sprigs fresh dill, chopped
¼	c. chopped pecans
½	tsp. sea salt
½	bunch fresh mint, chopped
	juice of 1 small lemon
1	bunch large-leaf spinach, washed and trimmed

Instructions

For lentil salad

Mix together lentils, peppers, onion, garlic, and bay leaf. In a large pan, heat olive oil at medium–high heat. When pan is hot, pour lentil mixture in pan, and cover with 5 cups water. Add sea salt, and turn heat back up to high. When water reaches a boil, turn heat back down to medium, and let simmer uncovered for 20 minutes or until lentils are soft but firm.

Drain lentils, and place in a large bowl. Toss in lemon juice and parsley, and let cool. Serve at room temperature.

For sunchokes

Preheat oven to 450 degrees. In a bowl, combine sunchokes, olive oil, and sea salt. Spread mixture onto a large baking sheet, and place in oven on middle rack. Cook for 10 minutes, then toss sunchokes and return to oven for another 10 minutes. When cooked, take sunchokes out of oven, and let cool before serving.

For dolmas

Cook brown rice and set aside.

In a large pan, heat olive oil at medium heat. Add onion, garlic, parsley, dill, pecans, and sea salt, and sauté until onions become transparent. Add brown rice, and sauté for 5 minutes. Take off heat, and let cool. Once cool, add mint and lemon juice to mixture.

In a large pot, steam spinach until leaves are completely wilted. Take off heat.

Lay out 4 or 5 spinach leaves flat on work surface, layered on top of each other to make a 4-inch diameter circle. Place 1 heaping tbsp. of rice mixture in the middle of circle, and roll spinach to enfold, tucking in edges as you go. If needed, add more spinach to keep rice from falling out. Continue until all leaves are used. Place completed dolmas, tightly lined up next to each other, in a container. When finished, drizzle a couple tbsp. olive oil over dolmas, cover, and refrigerate. Recipe makes roughly 10 dolmas.

SPLIT YELLOW MOONG DAL WITH
CASHEW CREAM RAITA AND GREEN SALAD

This Indian lentil soup is vividly colorful with a mild spice.

Serves 2

Ingredients

Dal

   1 c. split yellow moong beans
   1 tbsp. coconut oil
   1 tsp. cumin seeds
   1 1-inch piece of ginger, peeled and finely chopped
   4 c. water
      pinch of turmeric
   1 tsp. ground coriander
      sea salt to taste
   1 sprig of cilantro, finely chopped

Raita

   1 cashew cream recipe
   ½ c. cucumber, peeled, seeded, and finely chopped
   1 scallion, thinly sliced
      pinch of cumin
      pinch of coriander
      juice from ¼ lime
   1 tsp. apple cider vinegar
      sea salt to taste

      green salad

Instructions

For dal

Soak moong beans for 10 minutes. Then strain, rinse, and
set aside.

   Heat the oil in a large saucepan over medium heat for 1
minute. Add cumin seeds. When seeds begin to sputter, add the
ginger and stir, making sure cumin seeds and ginger don't burn.

Add moong beans to pan. Cook for 2 to 3 minutes, stirring constantly. Then add the water. Stir in turmeric, coriander, and sea salt. When soup begins to bubble, reduce the heat to medium low and simmer for 40 minutes, stirring occasionally. If dal thickens too quickly, add a little water to the pan. Remove the pan from the heat when the beans are soft.

For raita
Combine all ingredients in a bowl. You're done!

To serve, sprinkle dal with fresh cilantro and a dollop of raita, with green salad as a side.

CHICKEN CABBAGE WRAPS
WITH SESAME SUGAR SNAP PEAS
One of my favorite easy crunchy lunches.
   Serves 2

Ingredients

Filling
- 1 tbsp. sesame oil
- 2 boneless chicken breasts, chopped into small cubes and lightly sea salted
- 1 carrot, finely chopped
- 1 celery stalk, finely chopped
- ¼ head of red cabbage, thinly sliced
   sea salt to taste
- 4 large Napa cabbage leaves
   lime wedges

Sauce
- ¼ c. almond butter
- ¼ c. water
- 1 tsp. soy sauce
- 1 tsp. sesame oil
- ½ tsp. apple cider vinegar

½ tsp. maple syrup
   juice from ¼ lime

Add-ons
¼ c. basil, finely chopped
¼ c. cilantro, finely chopped
¼ c. mint, finely chopped
1 mango, thinly sliced
4 lime wedges
1 tbsp. crushed almonds

Sugar Snap Peas
2 c. sugar snap peas
1 tbsp. sesame oil
   sea salt
½ tsp. sesame seeds

Instructions
In a large pan, heat sesame oil at medium-high heat. Place chicken into pan, and sauté for 2 minutes, until outside of chicken turns white. Add carrots, celery, red cabbage, and cover, turning heat to medium. Keep covered for 5 minutes, stirring occasionally, then remove from heat.

When ready to serve, place a few spoonfuls inside a Napa cabbage leaf (2 per person), and squeeze fresh lime over chicken. Top with sauce and add-ons of choice.

For sauce
In a small bowl, combine almond butter and water to reach smooth consistency. Add all other ingredients and stir to combine.

For sugar snap peas
Steam peas for 1 minute, until they become bright green. Then place in a bowl, drizzle with sesame oil and sea salt to taste, and sprinkle sesame seeds over for a finishing touch.

MEZZE—QUINOA TABOULI, HUMMUS, AND TAHINI

Tabouli is traditionally made with bulgur wheat. This gluten-free alternative has its own nutty flavor and is also packed with protein.

Serves 2

Ingredients

Tabouli

- 1 c. quinoa
- 2 c. water
- pinch of sea salt
- 1½ c. grape tomatoes
- 1 bunch parsley, coarsely chopped
- ½ bunch mint, coarsely chopped
- juice from ½ a lemon
- 2 tbsp. olive oil
- sea salt to taste

Hummus

- juice from 1 lemon
- ¼ c. sesame tahini paste
- 1 garlic clove, minced
- 2 tbsp. olive oil
- 1 tsp. sea salt
- ½ tsp. cumin
- 1 15-oz. can garbanzo beans, thoroughly rinsed
- water, as needed
- pinch of paprika

Tahini Sauce

- ½ c. sesame tahini paste
- ¼ c. water
- juice from ¼ lemon
- ¼ tsp. sea salt
- ½ tsp. olive oil

gluten-free flatbread

Instructions

For tabouli
Place quinoa, water, and pinch of salt in a small pot, and
bring to boil. Cover, reduce heat to medium low, and simmer
until fully cooked. Remove from heat and let cool to room
temperature. Once cooled, toss all ingredients together in a
large bowl, and salt to taste.

For hummus
In a food processor, combine lemon juice and tahini until
smooth. Add garlic, olive oil, sea salt, and cumin, and blend for
1 minute. Add garbanzo beans in three segments, adding water
as needed to achieve desired consistency. (If using a blender,
more water will be needed.) When smooth, pour into a bowl,
sprinkle with a pinch of paprika, drizzle olive oil, and serve.

For tahini
In a small bowl, stir together tahini and water until mixture
becomes light in color and smooth in texture. Add lemon juice,
sea salt, and olive oil, and stir to combine. Done!

Serve all with gluten-free flatbread.

MUSHROOM FRITTATA WITH COLORFUL ROOT VEGETABLE SALAD
Mushrooms are earthy, meaty, and rich in flavor.
Serves 4

Ingredients

Frittata
- 6 eggs
- 1 tbsp. water
- ½ tsp. sea salt
- 2 tbsp. olive oil
- 3½ oz. mushrooms of choice (shiitake or white work well)

6 scallions

¼ c. sun-dried tomato, thinly sliced

freshly ground black pepper, to taste

Root Vegetable Salad

1 large carrot, shredded

1 large beet, shredded

½ head radicchio, thinly sliced

1 tbsp. olive oil

1 tbsp. balsamic vinegar

sea salt and pepper to taste

Instructions

Preheat oven to 350 degrees.

In a small bowl, beat eggs with 1 tbsp. water and sea salt. Set aside.

Heat olive oil in a small frying pan at medium-high heat. Add mushrooms, scallions, and sun-dried tomato, and toss for 5 minutes. Pour egg mixture into pan and stir continuously for 1 minute. Then cook for 5 more minutes on stove, smoothing any air bubbles that form.

Place pan in oven on middle rack and cook for 12 to 15 minutes, until top of frittata is golden brown.

For the root vegetable salad

Mix all ingredients in a bowl. Done!

RICE VERMICELLI WITH SHREDDED VEGETABLES, SESAME, SEAWEED, AND TOFU OR TILAPIA

Exotic, sensual, and aromatic, this dish is nutrient rich, delicious, and filling.

Serves 2

Ingredients

- 4 oz. rice vermicelli noodles
- 1 medium carrot, peeled into long strands with a vegetable peeler
- 1 small zucchini, peeled into long strands with a vegetable peeler
- 1 oz. arame seaweed, soaked in water for 10 minutes and drained
- 2 stalks celery, finely chopped
- 1 tbsp. sesame oil
- 7 oz. extra-firm tofu or ½ lb. tilapia fillet
   sesame seeds

Dressing
- 2 tbsp. sesame oil
- 2 tbsp. soy sauce
- 2 tbsp. rice vinegar
- 1 1-inch piece fresh ginger, minced

Instructions

To make dressing, combine all ingredients in a small bowl. Set aside.

Place noodles in a large pot of boiling water and boil for 3 minutes. Rinse, strain, and pour into a large bowl. Toss with dressing. Toss in carrot, zucchini, seaweed, and celery.

To cook the tofu or fish, in a small pan, heat 1 tbsp. sesame oil at medium–high heat. Add protein choice and sauté until it begins to brown, about 5 minutes. When cooked, add to bowl and toss to combine. Sprinkle with sesame seeds before serving.

DINNER

PASTA MARINARA WITH KALE AND FENNEL SALAD

The salty taste of this delicious pasta pairs perfectly with the crunchy salad.

   Serves 4

Ingredients

2	tsp. olive oil
1	clove garlic, minced
13½	oz. tomato puree
½	tsp. sea salt
1	can tuna, packed in olive oil
½	c. fresh basil
½	c. fresh parsley
8	oz. quinoa pasta shells or whole wheat pasta shells

Salad

1	bunch kale, ripped into medium pieces
1	fennel bulb, finely sliced
1	tbsp. olive oil
2	tbsp. balsamic vinegar
	sea salt and pepper to taste

Instructions

In a small pot, heat 1 tsp. olive oil at medium heat. Add garlic and sauté until transparent. Pour in tomato purée and stir. When sauce begins to boil, turn heat to medium low, drizzle with 1 tsp. olive oil and sea salt, and cover. Simmer for 30 minutes, stirring occasionally. Add tuna, fresh basil, and parsley to tomato sauce.

   While sauce simmers, boil pasta in a large pot to desired firmness. Drain and pour back into pot. Add ½ of tomato sauce to pasta. Serve, spooning reserved tomato sauce on top.

For salad

Place kale in a large salad bowl. Sprinkle with sea salt and massage until kale becomes bright green and wilted. Add fennel.

Drizzle over olive oil and balsamic vinegar, and toss to combine. Add sea salt and pepper to taste, and you're done!

ROAST CHICKEN WITH ARUGULA AND ARTICHOKES

Brining the chicken before cooking it ensures insanely moist and delicious meat. This is optional, but recommended.

Serves 4

Ingredients

- 1 whole chicken, 3 to 4 lbs.
- 1 lemon, halved
- 1 onion, quartered
- 1 head garlic, separated and unpeeled
    a few sprigs thyme, rosemary, and/or tarragon
    bacon (optional)
- 1 tbsp. olive oil
- 1 tsp. sea salt
- 2 bunches arugula
- 4 artichokes

Dressing

- 8 tsp. olive oil
    juice of 1 lemon
- 2 tsp. tahini
- 2 tsp. honey
    sea salt and pepper to taste

Instructions

To brine chicken

Fill a large pot with water, and add ¾ cup sea salt and ¾ cup sugar. Stir to dissolve. Place the chicken in the pot, making sure water covers the chicken, and refrigerate. This can be done a few hours before cooking but can also be done overnight. When ready to cook, remove chicken from brine.

For chicken

Preheat oven to 475 degrees.

Place chicken in a deep roasting pan. Stuff with lemon, onion, garlic, and herbs. If desired, stuff a few strips of bacon under the skin of the bird. This adds flavor and crispiness.

Rub olive oil and sea salt all over the skin of the chicken to coat, and place in the oven. Cook for about 1 hour, until the outside is golden brown and crispy and the meat is fully cooked. If the chicken looks dry while roasting, add a few spoonfuls of water to the pot. Once cooked, remove from oven, and let cool on stovetop. Do not cut open the chicken until it's ready to be served; it will keep cooking in its juices after removed from the oven.

For arugula

Place arugula in a large salad bowl. Drizzle with olive oil, squeeze half a lemon over, and toss. Add sea salt and pepper to taste.

For artichokes

To trim artichokes, remove any outside leaves that are brown, cut the stems to about a quarter-inch length, and cut the top third of the artichokes off so that the artichoke hearts are barely visible. Place artichokes face down in a steaming basket, and steam for 20 minutes or until soft. Remove from heat, and let cool to room temperature.

Mix dressing ingredients in a small bowl. Serve artichokes with dressing.

RED CURRY WITH VEGETABLES
AND BROWN BASMATI RICE

I love the aroma of a good curry, and it's a great way to eat rice and vegetables.

Serves 4

Ingredients

1½ c. brown basmati rice, rinsed and drained

1 tbsp. coconut oil

1 onion, chopped into large pieces

2 garlic cloves, minced

1 tbsp. freshly grated ginger

2 carrots, chopped into large pieces

2 stalks celery, chopped

½ tsp. salt

1 13½-oz. can tomato puree

1 13½-oz. can coconut milk

1 tbsp. red curry paste

10 basil leaves

Suggested Add-ins

1 head broccoli, cut into pieces

2 c. cauliflower pieces

2 c. cabbage, red or green, chopped

1 c. bok choy or dark leafy greens, chopped

Instructions

Cook rice according to directions on package and set aside.

While rice cooks, prepare curry. In a large pot, heat coconut oil at medium-high heat. Add in onion, garlic, ginger, carrots, celery, and salt, and sauté for 2 minutes. Pour in tomato purée. When sauce begins to bubble, stir in coconut milk and red curry paste. Turn heat to medium low, cover, and simmer for 15 minutes, stirring occasionally. Toss preferred vegetables into pot, stir, and cover pot again. Cook curry another 10 minutes. If adding dark leafy greens, including basil leaves, wait to add them until the very end.

Serve over rice.

QUINOA CROQUETTES WITH BUTTERNUT SQUASH AND RADISHES

These filling pancakes are packed with a completely vegetarian source of protein.

Serves 4

Ingredients

     1 c. quinoa, cooked and cooled to room temperature
     4 eggs, beaten
     ½ tsp. salt
     1 tsp. cumin
     1 tsp. cinnamon
     ½ tsp. chili powder (optional)
     1 onion, chopped
     2 garlic cloves, minced
     1 c. breadcrumbs
        water, if needed
     7 tsp. olive oil, divided into 2 tbsp. for croquettes,
        1 tsp. for squash
     1 bunch radishes, quartered, greens trimmed and reserved
     1 butternut squash, skin and seeds removed,
        chopped into small cubes

Instructions

For croquettes

In a large bowl, combine quinoa, eggs, salt, cumin, cinnamon, and chili powder. Stir in onion, garlic, and breadcrumbs, and let sit for a few minutes to allow breadcrumbs to soak up moisture. Using your hands, form mixture into small patties, adding more breadcrumbs or water if necessary.

Heat the olive oil in a large pan over medium heat. Add patties to pan and cook on each side for 8 to 10 minutes, until outsides are brown.

For squash and radishes

In a separate pan, heat olive oil at medium-high heat, and toss in radishes and squash, sprinkling with salt. Sauté until outsides begin to brown and squash becomes soft. Add in radish greens, cover pan, and turn heat down to medium. Keep covered for 2 minutes to allow greens to wilt. Uncover and remove from heat.

PAN-ROASTED SALMON WITH ROASTED POTATOES AND MUSTARD DILL DRESSING

This so-easy recipe will wow your friends and family.

Serves 4

Ingredients

12	Red Bliss potatoes, cut into quarters
	salt
	pepper
2	tbsp. olive oil
1	tsp. caraway seeds
4	salmon fillets

Sauce

½	c. plain yogurt
¼	c. finely chopped fresh dill
1	tbsp. full-grain mustard

Instructions

Preheat oven to 450 degrees.

Toss potatoes to coat with salt, pepper, oil, and caraway seeds. Place on a large baking sheet and roast until cooked through and brown on outside, about 30 minutes.

Coat salmon fillets lightly with salt.

Heat a large pan at medium-high heat. Place fillets in pan and cook uncovered for 5 minutes. Flip fillets over to other side and cover. Cook for another 5 minutes. To check if salmon is cooked, pull apart and check the middle: meat should be opaque and soft, while outside will be brown and crispy. Remove from heat and serve with potatoes, dill sauce, and a green salad.

SUSHI BOWL—SEARED TUNA WITH SUSHI RICE, DAIKON, GINGER, WATERCRESS, AND AVOCADO

This complete meal contains pungent and bitter tastes, paired with the sweet rice and tuna.

Serves 4

Ingredients

  1   c. sushi rice

1¼ c. water

  ¼ c. rice vinegar

  2 tsp. honey

  1 tsp. grapeseed oil or vegetable oil

     pinch of sea salt

  4 tuna fillets, ¼ pound each

  4 tsp. sesame oil, divided into ½ tsp. for each fillet, 2 tsp. for greens

     sea salt

  1 1-inch piece fresh ginger, peeled and finely grated

  1 bunch watercress

  1 daikon radish, peeled into long strips

  1 avocado, divided into quarters

     sesame seeds

     nori sheets

Instructions

Rinse rice and place in pot with water. Bring water to boil, cover rice, and turn heat to medium low. Simmer for 15 minutes. Turn heat off but keep rice covered for another 10 minutes to allow water to be absorbed.

In a small bowl, combine rice vinegar, honey, and grapeseed oil. Stir until honey dissolves. Stir into rice, adding a pinch of sea salt, and set aside.

Coat tuna fillets with sesame oil, and lightly dust with sea salt.

Heat a large pan at medium-high heat. Place fillets in pan and cook uncovered for 5 minutes. Flip fillets over to other side and cover. Cook for another 5 minutes. To check if tuna is cooked, pull apart and check the middle: meat should be opaque and soft, while outside will be brown and crispy. Remove from heat and set aside.

In a separate pan, heat sesame oil at medium heat. Toss in grated ginger and sauté for 1 minute. Add in watercress and sauté until greens wilt. Sprinkle with sea salt.

To serve, place 1 tuna fillet over sushi rice, with greens, daikon, and ¼ avocado. Top with sesame seeds. Use the nori sheets to roll the ingredients together in sushi rolls, if preferred.

BAKED POTATO WITH MUSHROOMS, LEEKS, AND RAINBOW SWISS CHARD

Potatoes offer a filling alternative to gluten-filled grains.

Serves 4

Ingredients

- 4 potatoes, scrubbed
- 2 tsp. olive oil, divided into 1 tsp. for potatoes, 1 tsp. for mushroom mixture

  sea salt
- 4 portobello mushrooms, stems removed, washed, and diced
- 2 leeks, thinly sliced
- 2 tbsp. balsamic vinegar
- 1 bunch rainbow chard, thinly sliced

  sea salt and pepper to taste

  cashew cream (optional)

Instructions

Preheat oven to 350 degrees.

Puncture each potato several times all over with a fork. Lightly coat potatoes with olive oil, sprinkle with sea salt, and place on middle rack in oven. Bake for 1 hour, then test for softness. Potatoes may need more time, depending on the oven. When cooked through, remove from the oven and set aside.

While potatoes bake, prepare mushrooms, leeks, and chard. In a large pan, heat 1 tsp. olive oil at medium-high heat, then toss in mushrooms and leeks. Sprinkle with sea salt and sauté for 2 minutes. Once mushrooms and leeks begin to soften, pour in balsamic vinegar to mixture and continue cooking, stirring occasionally, until mushrooms are reduced to half their size and leeks are fully softened. Add rainbow chard to pan, turn heat to medium low, and cover for 2 minutes to allow chard to wilt. Add sea salt and pepper to taste and set aside.

On each plate, put a potato, sliced down the middle and opened, and add a portion of the mushroom mixture on top. If desired, put a dollop of cashew cream on top.

SNACKS

A piece of fresh fruit, cut vegetables, or a homemade trail mix are perfect go-to snacks. Here are some other options that you may enjoy.

SAVORY ROASTED NUTS

An easy and healthy snack to put in your purse when you're on the go.
8 servings

Ingredients

- 1 tsp. garlic powder
- 1 tsp. paprika
- 1 tsp. cumin
- ⅓ c. maple syrup
- 2 tbsp. applesauce
- 3 c. assorted nuts (almonds, cashews, and pecans work well)
- 2 tsp. olive oil
- salt

Instructions

Preheat oven to 350 degrees.

Combine garlic powder, paprika, cumin, maple syrup, and applesauce in a bowl. Toss in nuts and olive oil, and mix to coat completely. Spread out nuts evenly on a baking sheet, and sprinkle with salt. Place in oven and cook for 10 minutes. Toss and return to oven another 15 minutes or until nuts are golden brown. Remove from oven and cool completely.

SUNFLOWER AND KALAMATA PÂTÉ
A unique spread, perfect for entertaining friends.
16 servings

Ingredients
- 1   c. sunflower seeds, soaked at least 4 hours (can be soaked overnight)
- 1   garlic clove, chopped
  juice from ¼ lemon
- ½   tsp. olive oil
- 1   tsp. capers, with additional ½ tsp. caper juice (can substitute for ½ tsp. salt)
- 10   Kalamata olives, pits removed

Instructions
Place seeds and garlic in a blender and blend, adding water until pâté becomes smooth and thick. Add lemon juice, olive oil, capers, and olives, and continue blending until fully incorporated. Serve with sliced vegetables or gluten-free crackers.

ENERGY BARS WITH DRIED FRUIT AND OATS
Your own homemade energy bar.
Makes 8 bars

Ingredients
- 1   c. oats
- ½   tsp. sea salt
- ½   tsp. cinnamon
- 1   banana
- ⅓   c. maple syrup
- 1   c. almond butter
- ⅓   c. applesauce
- 1   tbsp. coconut flakes
- 1   tbsp. chia seeds
- ⅓   c. sunflower seeds
- ⅓   c. almonds
- ½   c. dried fruit (apricots, raisins, cranberries, cherries)

Instructions

Preheat oven to 350 degrees.

Combine all ingredients in a bowl. Pour mixture into an 8-x-8-inch square baking pan and smooth to evenly distribute. Mixture will be about 1 to 1½ inches thick. Place on middle rack of oven and bake for 30 to 40 minutes, until top becomes golden brown.

Remove from oven and cool completely in pan. Cover with aluminum foil and refrigerate overnight. To serve, slice into bars and wrap individually in plastic wrap. Keep refrigerated or in the freezer for up to one month.

PUMPKIN MUFFINS WITH THYME AND PECANS

These bake-ahead treats are gluten-free and delicious.

Ingredients

Dry Ingredients

    1   c. all-purpose gluten-free flour

    ⅓ c. organic coconut flour

    ½ c. almond flour

    ½ c. tapioca starch

 1½ tsp. baking powder

    1   tsp. baking soda

    ½ tsp. sea salt

    1   tsp. xanthan gum powder

    1   tsp. ground cinnamon

    2   tsp. dried thyme

    ½ c. roughly chopped pecans

Wet Ingredients

    ¾ c. maple syrup

    1   c. pumpkin puree

    ⅓ c. coconut oil, melted

    2   eggs, beaten

    1   tbsp. vanilla extract

    ½ tsp. lemon juice

    ½ c. coconut milk

Instructions

Preheat oven to 350 degrees.

Grease a 12-muffin tin with coconut oil.

In a large bowl, whisk together all of the dry ingredients.
In a separate bowl, combine the wet ingredients, then add
to dry mixture, beating to incorporate. If batter needs a little
more liquid, add up to ¼ cup coconut milk, until it reaches a
smooth consistency. Stir in chopped pecans.

Spoon the batter into 12 muffin cups, filling them close to
the top. Bake until domed and golden: roughly 20 to 25 minutes,
depending on the oven. If a wooden toothpick inserted into the
center comes out clean, they're done.

Cool on a wire rack. Remove the muffins from the pan
after five minutes, and allow them to continue cooling on
the rack. This helps to keep their bottoms from getting soggy.
Wrap and freeze leftover muffins in freezer bags.

SWEET AND SALTY AVOCADO HALVES

A creamy and simple snack that satisfies.

Serves 1

Ingredients

  1 stalk celery, finely chopped
  ½ avocado
  ½ tsp. olive oil
  ½ tsp. honey
     sea salt
     pepper

Place celery inside the seed indent of the avocado half. Drizzle
with olive oil and honey, and sprinkle with sea salt and pepper.
Done!

CALIFORNIA RICE BALLS

Try each of the flavors for these easy snacks.

Serves 2: 2 rice balls each

Ingredients

    1 c. sushi rice, rinsed
    1¼ c. water
    ½ tsp. sesame seeds
    2 nori seaweed sheets

Filling options

    1 tbsp. of any of the following:
        smoked salmon
        chopped peanuts
        avocado, diced
        cucumber, peeled, seeded, and finely chopped
        carrot, finely chopped
        umeboshi plum paste

Instructions

Pour rice and water in a small pot and bring to boil. Cover rice and simmer for 15 minutes, then turn off heat but keep covered another 10 minutes. Allow rice to cool completely.

Once rice has cooled, gather by the handful and form a ball. Make an indent in one side and fill rice ball with a spoonful of desired filling. Sprinkle sesame seeds and wrap with a nori sheet.

SENSUOUS GREEN SMOOTHIE

Get your greens any time of the day with this delicious fruity smoothie.

Serves 1

Ingredients

    ½ banana
    1 c. fruit (berries, tropical fruits, or even veggies like pumpkin and squash work well)

    1 tbsp. nut butter
    ½ c. chopped greens
   1½ c. water, coconut water, or almond milk

Add-ins (let the amount be guided by your desire)
        cinnamon
        nutmeg
        raw cacao powder
        maca powder
        coconut manna (coconut butter)
    ¼ avocado
    ¼ c. yogurt
        spirulina
        chia seeds

Instructions

Place all base ingredients in a blender and blend until
smooth. Once you have your base, choose add-ins and add
small spoonfuls to taste. Blend again until fully combined.
Add more liquid if you desire a thinner smoothie.

DESSERT

BALSAMIC STRAWBERRIES WITH CASHEW CREAM

This dessert hits both sweet and sour notes, with one of my
favorite sensuous fruits.
    Serves 4

Ingredients

   16 oz. strawberries, cut into thick slices
    2 tsp. balsamic vinegar
    2 tsp. honey
    2 twists fresh black pepper
       cashew cream

Instructions

Combine strawberries, vinegar, honey, and pepper in a medium
bowl. Let sit at room temperature for at least 15 minutes.
Divide among 4 bowls, and spoon a dollop of cashew cream
on top. Serve.

RAW MACAROONS:
VANILLA LEMON AND CURRY CACAO

Coconut manna is the ground flesh of the coconut and is a
fabulous base for desserts, smoothies, and snacks.

Makes 6 to 8, 2 per serving

Ingredients

Base

- 1 c. shredded coconut
- 2 tbsp. maple syrup
- 2 tbsp. coconut manna, softened
-    pinch of sea salt

Vanilla Lemon

- 1 tsp. vanilla extract
-    zest from ½ lemon

Curry Cacao

- 2 tsp. raw cacao powder
-    large pinch of curry powder

Instructions

Mix all base ingredients together in a bowl until combined.
Then add ingredients for your flavor of choice. When mix is
fully combined and sticky, scoop heaping tablespoons into
your hands and roll into balls. One batch will make about 6 to
8 macaroons. Place in the refrigerator for at least 20 minutes
before serving.

THE CUPCAKE THAT DOES IT ALL

This mini gluten-free red velvet cupcake leaves packaged cupcakes in the dust.

Makes 2 dozen, 1 per serving

Ingredients

Dry Ingredients

¼ c. coconut flour

¼ c. all-purpose gluten-free flour

2 tbsp. raw cacao powder

¼ tsp. baking soda

¼ tsp. salt

Wet Ingredients

4 eggs, beaten

2 tbsp. coconut oil (melted) or grapeseed oil

½ c. maple syrup

4 tubes red food-coloring gel

Frosting

2 tsp. maple syrup

1 cashew cream recipe

Instructions

Preheat oven to 350 degrees.

Line one mini-muffin tin with mini cupcake wrappers or grease with oil. Set aside.

Whisk together dry ingredients in a large bowl. In a separate bowl, beat together wet ingredients until smooth. Gradually add the wet ingredients to the dry mixture, and beat to fully incorporate. Divide batter among cupcake wrappers, and bake for about 12 to 15 minutes or until a toothpick inserted in the middle comes out clean. Let cupcakes cool completely before frosting.

For frosting, stir maple syrup into cashew cream and refrigerate to set for at least 20 minutes before decorating cupcakes.

PARFAIT WITH CASHEW CREAM, CAKE HUNKS, AND TOASTED SWEET SEEDS

This dessert uses the cupcake recipe above in a different way.

Ingredients

For each parfait

2   cupcakes (see recipe above) broken into pieces and divided

1   cashew cream recipe, divided in 4 parts

1   c. raspberries, divided in 3 parts

Toasted sweet seeds

⅛   c. sliced almonds

⅛   c. chopped pecans

⅛   c. sunflower seeds

¼   tsp. cinnamon

pinch of sea salt

Instructions

In a small bowl, combine nuts, sunflower seeds, cinnamon, and sea salt. Pour into a medium pan, set at medium heat, and toast until nuts become fragrant and begin to brown. Set aside.

Place one cupcake (broken up into pieces) into the bottom of a mason jar or a medium-sized drinking glass. Layer one quarter of cashew cream on top. Then layer with half of the toasted nuts. Top with ⅓ c. raspberries, and then cover with another quarter of cashew cream. Repeat layers: cake, cashew cream, nuts, raspberries, cashew cream. Add last layer of berries on top. Refrigerate for at least 1 hour to set.

REFRESHING FRUIT SALAD
WITH FRESH HERBS AND FLOWERS

The herbs and flowers make this fruit salad savory and memorable.
Serves 4

Ingredients

         1   pink grapefruit
         1   navel orange
         1   c. pineapple
         2   kiwis
        ½   cucumber
             juice from ½ lime
         2   tbsp. coconut milk
         1   sprig fresh cilantro, chopped
  2 or 3   mint leaves, chopped
         1   c. edible flowers (nasturtium, pansies, etc.)

Instructions

Peel all of the fruit, chop each into 1-inch chunks, and toss
together in a bowl. Add lime juice and coconut milk and
toss. Toss in fresh herbs last. Can be served immediately but is
best if refrigerated for at least a half-hour to let the flavors set.
Before serving, top with flowers.

ALMOND, CHERRY, AND CACAO TRUFFLES

Mouth-watering truffles will satisfy your chocolate craving.
Makes 8 to 10, 2 per serving

Ingredients

        ⅓   c. almond butter
         2   tbsp. maple syrup
         1   tsp. coconut flour
         2   tbsp. cacao powder
             pinch of sea salt
        ¼   c. dried cherries

Instructions

In a bowl, mix together almond butter, maple syrup, coconut flour, cacao powder, and sea salt until blended and smooth. In another bowl, pour a few spoonfuls of cacao powder and set aside.

Take one cherry and use a heaping teaspoon of almond mixture to envelope the cherry. Roll into a ball with hands and then roll in bowl of cacao to coat the outside. Repeat until all of mixture has been used. This will make about 8 to 10 truffles. Place in a closed container and refrigerate.

DARK CHOCOLATE–COVERED KUMQUATS

Bittersweet and tangy, these kumquats are a perfect way to end a special meal.

Makes 20, 2 per serving

Ingredients

- ⅓ cup pitted dates
- ½ cup almond milk
-    pinch of cinnamon
-    pinch of cayenne pepper (optional)
- 1 oz. unsweetened baking chocolate
- 20 kumquats (leave peel on)

Instructions

Line a large plate with wax paper and set aside.

Blend dates and almond milk in a blender until smooth. Pour into a saucepan and bring to a boil, adding cinnamon and cayenne. Reduce to a simmer and continue to cook while stirring over a low flame for 5 to 10 minutes, until thickened. Remove from the heat and stir in the chocolate until completely melted.

Dip kumquats to partially cover. Set dipped pieces on wax paper and refrigerate for at least 30 minutes to set.

Your body, absolutely unique and like no other, configured like
no other in its proportions, has its unique movement that
belongs entirely to you. You are connected to your body.
Your body is connected to your movement. Allow your
movement to connect you into your life.

SERA SOLSTICE

10 The Secrets of Pleasurable Movement

OUR CULTURE'S PREVAILING assumption is that the way to
lose weight and tone your body is to push it to extremes that
feel punishing. Just consider the rise in popularity of boot camps,
extreme spinning, and other fitness regimes where you are yelled
at to keep going. Rarely do we think of exercise as a source of
pleasure. For many women who know they should be exercising,
exercise often and easily falls by the wayside in favor of other pri-
orities. I can't tell you that moving your body is optional if you
want to tone your body and lose weight, but I can tell you that
there is definitely a more feminine approach. It's time to have a
closer look at your beliefs about movement, shed old-paradigm
thinking, and embrace the new standard of pleasurable movement.
Let's first examine some of the common cultural misconceptions
about exercise that you may have accepted as true.

Your animal doesn't want to be punished or bored. If your
approach to moving your body is punishing and boring, it will
only be a matter of time until your animal rebels. And when she
does, you'll feel guilty about ditching your exercise program. But

you'll ditch it all the same because punishing yourself is simply not sustainable. I'm not alone in my thinking. A recent article in the *New York Times* showed that people's attitudes toward physical activity influence whether they lose weight. A study showed that people who were told that they were walking one mile for pleasure ate less and made healthier food choices afterward compared to those who were told that they were walking for exercise. The pleasure reaped from the experience was a reward unto itself, so the walkers in that group didn't feel the need to compensate for a punishing experience with food.

My last foray with punishing exercise was more than ten years ago, when I went to a nearby gym in a moment of feeling disgusted by my body and paid in full for a yearlong membership. I went once the following week, disliked the ambience, and never went again.

In the punishing paradigm, we're led to think of working out as a mechanical process that burns calories and, therefore, fat. Something as subjective as ambience is not taken into consideration. The message we absorb about exercise is that if our bodies don't like the way we are pushing them, it's too bad. Your animal isn't supposed to enjoy it, just endure it. With this mentality, exercise is reduced to a clinical function stripped of all poetry and pleasure. Compared to the enjoyment the mind can provide, it's no wonder so many women find working out boring.

However, the dirty little secret of the workout world is that there is a significant cost to compromising the pleasure and enjoyment you could have moving your body. When you push yourself to do exercise your animal doesn't enjoy, you trigger a self-created stress response, in which calorie-burning efficiency is decreased and fat storage is encouraged. By triggering a stress response, the same exercise that was intended to make you lose weight can cause you to gain it. That's why many women who toil away on the treadmill or StairMaster at the gym find themselves not losing a pound—or they get so bored they never go back! Instead of fixating on any one particular fitness program, the real goal is to make movement an enjoyable part of your daily lifestyle.

The second point to remember is that when it comes to weight loss, your metabolism influences your success more than the calories-in-calories-out equation. Your metabolic rate is directly influenced by relaxation. So why would you ever want to make a practice of exercise that stresses you out, especially in the name of weight loss? The rewards for doing exercise the right way, in pleasure, are many. Pleasurable exercise stimulates a reduction in cortisol levels and a release of endorphins that create a feeling of euphoria. The so-called runner's high can be accomplished through any form of exercise your body enjoys.

It has gotten to the point where women are tired and disillusioned with the punishing methods of losing weight, and they are clamoring for something more, something different. But the message we've received is that if we want to change our shape, the only way is the punishing way. Not only is this untrue, but it is unsustainable. Thankfully, there is a more feminine and enjoyable way to exercise that can enliven your soul, create a deeper relationship with your animal, and lead to physical change. Instead of punishing exercise, I advocate for pleasurable movement.

THE ART OF PLEASURABLE MOVEMENT

The truth is, all animals take pleasure in moving. What makes a form of movement punishing or pleasurable is not the specifics of the movement itself but the attitude with which it is performed. Punishing movement is done to the body, while pleasurable movement is done with the body. Horse whisperer Ray Hunt describes an analogous mind-set when he works with horses: "It's the life in his body I'm trying to work with. It's the harmony. It's the rhythms. It's like dancing with someone."

I remember watching movies about horses when I was growing up and noticing that the jockeys always seemed to be brushing the horses. I later found out why. Brushing the horses relaxes them, and relaxed horses enjoy running fast. The same goes for you. When you change your perspective to move with your body, you will enjoy the experience and get the results you're looking for.

Pleasurable movement is not necessarily soft or gentle; your animal enjoys intensity, too. However, there's a big difference between what I refer to as an intense workout versus a punishing workout. In an intense workout, you can be panting, sweating, and feeling the burn of your muscles, but instead of biting your lip, clenching your teeth, and bemoaning how painful it is or checking out of the body altogether, you stay present with your breath and your sensations. If you are exercising with intensity and staying present with your sensations and breath, you may discover that the intense workout is not as painful as you thought it would be. It may even be pleasurable in a sweaty kind of way. However, if you don't stay present with the sensations of your body but check out to the recesses of your mind, you essentially abandon your body, so it will feel painful and punishing to her.

The ideal relationship with movement has specific qualities. It needs to be regular, have variety, and be pleasurable and fun. Sometimes this means getting out of your comfort zone and trying new things (including some of the recommendations I make later in the chapter). If you haven't exercised in a while, any movement that gets your heart rate up might initially feel strenuous. It will take some commitment to stay with whatever movement you choose. Looking for the activity that you think will burn the most calories in the least amount of time won't pro- vide long-term success if you don't enjoy it and stick with it. So, choose an activity that speaks to you, that ignites your curiosity, and that may even require courage.

WHAT IS YOUR ANIMAL'S PLEASURE?

If you want to love how your body looks, start being active in ways your body loves. Whatever gets you into your body in a way you enjoy constitutes pleasurable movement. It can be as simple as walking. Walking is a safe and easy way for women to start a habit of pleasurable movement. It is low impact, has no cost, and offers another powerful way to connect with your animal. Walking calms the mind, heightens creativity, and warms you up for other pleasurable movement practices. Relationship experts recommend taking a walk with your partner to establish better communication, and I suggest taking a walk with your animal so that you can strengthen your bond with her.

I recommend what fitness expert and samba dancer Theresa Stevens calls a "beauty walk." This is when you walk with attention to feeling beautiful and taking in the beauty of your environment. When you take a beauty walk, put your shoulders back, hold your head up high, and tune in to your natural sensu-ality. A daily beauty walk is a gift I encourage you to give yourself.

My client Erika refers to her beauty walk as "a sacred strut." Here's what she has to say about walking: "I was experiencing a deep heartache, and I could feel myself triggered into my old patterns of binging. But I checked in with my animal, and each time I felt the urge to binge, I walked out my door and down to the ocean's edge and stayed there until my energy shifted. No matter what was going on in my day, I gave myself this time to be, to pray, to relax into peace.

"I began walking an hour each night before bed. It was the relationship I had always dreamed of having with myself. It was ease over force, pleasure over stress, and it was available without any excuse. Every night I found myself in a walking meditation, in sacred connection with the universe, my body, and the power of my thoughts, breath, energy, and gratitude. As I walked, the layers of fear, hurt, pain, and judgment began to dissipate, and I emerged lighter, brighter, happier, more aware, and leaner than ever before. I lost twenty pounds that summer, but I gained so much more."

Whether it is gardening, tai chi, biking, team sports, or horsing around with your kids, when you move your body in ways that are fun, you invite your animal into a relaxed state where the magic of pleasurable weight loss takes place.

Mary Catherine, a fitness instructor from Los Angeles, was mis-erable when she heard me speak about the feminine approach to weight loss at a live conference. She had been using the masculine approach to weight loss and fitness, putting her animal through a grueling combination of extreme diets and punishing workouts. She told me, "Every time I show up at the gym, it is me against my body, punishing myself for not being good enough." Mary Catherine was approaching fitness the only way she knew how, pushing and grunting through the same workouts that she taught her clients. "My work environment is toxic. I don't know how to separate myself from my clients' bad body image, and it is only getting worse," she confessed to me. She was constantly fatigued, she had joint pain, her hair was falling out, her nails were brit-tle, she had stopped getting her period, and she was obsessively weighing herself a dozen times a day. All her efforts at self-control were reaching a breaking point. Feeling isolated and imprisoned, she often sat on her couch and cried. "If this is the way it's going to be, I don't want to go on," she told me.

When she heard my philosophy, Mary Catherine felt instantly relieved. "Just hearing the idea that a feminine approach existed made me feel lighter," she told me. "I assumed there were no other options for getting results than the hardcore workouts. I thought if you really want to lose weight, you need to suffer your way to it." I had Mary Catherine begin to work out in her apartment, with music and dance. She told me, "Working with my female body through dance made me just as sweaty as any gym workout. Except this time, instead of feeling punished, I truly had fun in the process."

PLEASURE PRACTICE
Your Movement Wish List

Write down all the different types of exercise you have tried and identify which felt pleasurable and which felt punishing. Now, write down what types of movement you haven't tried that sound pleasurable or intriguing to you. Be curious and creative.

PLEASURE BITE

Try a new form of movement you are attracted to, but with one important shift in attitude—imagine doing it *with* your animal instead of to your animal. Instead of resisting the sensations that come up during the movement as punishing, embrace the intensity of the movement by staying present with your animal's experience. Keep consciously breathing while you move.

USE PLEASURABLE MOVEMENT TO FEEL SEXY

We all want to feel sexy. Instead of having your sexiness be something that requires external validation, such as from your partner, the secret to feeling and being sexy is to find it inside yourself. And the secret for doing so is pleasurable, sensual movement. When you love the way your body moves, you'll feel relaxed, strong, free, and wild.

Pleasurable movement is an invitation to connect with the living, feeling, breathing part of you that desires to move joyfully, playfully, and sensually. It is reclamation of what feels good in your body, which will be different for everyone. You know you're moving pleasurably when you feel closer to yourself or when you're learning something about yourself. It may be the delicious joy of feeling yourself getting stronger or finding out that you have the capacity to do more than you thought was possible. Pleasurable movement is an invitation to be more of who you are and is an indispensable secret to unlocking your body wisdom.

At its heart, pleasurable movement is about sensuality. Theresa Stevens says, "Feeling sensual while you move is the secret sauce that makes all the difference in your motivation to add movement to your life every day because it feels amazing." What's more, we know that feeling sensual gets you to that coveted relaxation state. No matter the form of the movement itself, by having your attention on the sensuality of the experience, you will feel more connected with your animal and more motivated to continue. For example, I have female friends who tell me they feel sensual when they lift weights, and I believe them. I highly recommend a DVD called *Dance of the Kama Sutra* by Hemalayaa for learning sensual movement.

The idea of pleasurable movement ties into a bigger shift in the fitness world, where feminine alternatives to traditional workouts based in creativity, play, and mindfulness are increasingly popular. For example, Zumba is one of the pioneer modalities for reclaiming fun in movement, with its dance music, simple steps, and party atmosphere. Another is Shrink Session, a fitness program that mixes movement with affirmations, so that while you are moving your body, you are also setting intentions and reprogramming the beliefs of your ecology. These are only two of many innovative movement modalities that you can discover when you start to wade into the warm waters of pleasurable movement.

After one of my recent Pleasure Camps, one of the participants, Dina, gave me the following feedback: "I have to confess: although I am a health coach, I have always hated exercise. However, after being exposed to the teachings of pleasurable weight loss, I'm going to look at exercise with a new lens. Last night I went to Zumba, and the night before I went to a BodyFlow class, which is a combination of tai chi, yoga, and Pilates. Rather than muscling and grunting through it and worrying about keeping up with the right number of repetitions (the masculine, left-brain approach), I chose a feminine approach. I reframed exercise as movement and connected to the freedom of expression that comes with movement. I felt gratitude for this freedom, something I have taken for granted in the past. I let my belly hang out and decided not to worry about it. I honored my own limits, releasing the need to exercise perfectly. I made it playful and turned it all into a dance to express my authentic self. I connected to the possibility that if I move my body more, then perhaps I will become unstuck in other areas of my life. Most of all, I felt my body connect with Spirit. I could cry. I am now actually looking forward to future movement classes. This approach really works. Being in a tribe with other kindred spirits inspires and carries me more than ever."

Instead of moving in a linear way, sensual movement is also about using all your senses and finding the kind of natural movement that lives inside the power of the breasts and the hips. For example, in samba you run your fingers along your body while you dance, which connects you to your skin in a way that is sensual, playful, and fun.

PLEASURE BITE

Your female animal may be a fierce mountain lioness who loves intense movement. Be open to anything your animal loves, including movement that makes her feel wild and strong, like rock climbing, hiking, running, or biking on mountain trails.

THE POWER OF EMBODIMENT

One of the secrets of pleasurable weight loss is what is referred to as *embodiment.* When you are embodied, your awareness is in your body because you are fully grounded. In contrast, when you are doing things to the body or making decisions about the body, you are in the mind. When I am embodied, I feel like I am inhabiting my cells: I am fully present with and occupying my body. Embodiment is the most powerful tool we have for losing weight because we can only shift the body to where we would like it to go once we are fully present and inside of it. I feel the most embodied when I'm dancing. I'm able to release my mental preoccupations and be present with everything I am feeling. I connect with my heartbeat and my breath, the feeling of the dance in my feet, and how it affects my entire body.

Often when we want to lose weight, we start rationalizing with future thinking: "When I lose 20 pounds, I'm going to finally like the way my body looks." This kind of thinking takes us out of the body and into the head. In contrast, when you are embodied you'll feel, "I am here in this body and it feels good. I like this and I am happy to be here at my present weight."

Anything can get you embodied: dancing, walking, running, swimming, great conversation, meditation, passionate sex, hula hooping, or even being in nature. Eating a cookie or a plate of broccoli can make you feel embodied if you are fully present with all of your senses. Your ability to succeed with pleasurable weight loss hinges on discovering embodiment. Throughout the course of evolution, the creatures that have been the most successful are the ones who use their bodies to their fullest potential. They created their own niche in their ecosystem as they jumped, climbed, swam, and flew. Embodiment is a call to action to value being in your body by paying closer attention not only to what your animal wants but also to how she feels as she moves.

PLEASURE PRACTICE
What Movement Moves Your Soul?

What forms of movement seem most pleasurable to you? Write a list, and then seek out local classes, a community you can join, or take private lessons. Can you get your partner or a friend involved to make this even more sustainable? Women are communal creatures, and as you delve into pleasurable movement, it will be extremely helpful to be a part of a community that shares your same goal of having a more loving relationship with your body and reclaiming the pleasure of movement—the goal of the community can't simply be weight loss.

Another way to access pleasurable movement is by taking advantage of the proliferation of DVDs and online classes that are now available. I love the convenience of dance fitness DVDs, which allow me to learn from world-class instructors in the comfort of my home. Working out at home is a particularly feminine approach because it means we can fit movement into our schedules, before or after work, without ever leaving our nests.

MAKING TIME FOR MOVEMENT

It's easy to say you are too busy (aren't we all), but making time and space in your life for movement is non-negotiable if you want to have a happy animal. Imagine if your body were your romantic partner. If you filled your life with so many obligations and demands that you didn't have quality time for your beloved, your relationship would never flourish and would become at best a practical convenience. The same thing goes for your body. Movement is her quality time. If you say you don't have time for it, it's the same as telling your partner you don't have time. With any self-respect, your partner would not be happy as a low priority and would leave you. Your animal, however, short of death, can't leave you; she can only express her discontent and let you know something is wrong by gaining weight. Every time I notice myself rationalizing that I am too busy for movement, I remember this analogy, and it reminds me to stop taking my animal for granted.

What your body most wants is simple: she wants to feel alive. Yet sadly in our culture, this need is often neglected. You may let your mind come alive, allowing it to have a field day, exploring all kinds of stimulation, fun, and freedom, while you relegate only scraps of your attention to your body. As a result your mind feels like it is moving at a hundred miles a minute, and your body feels heavy and numb. Your struggle with weight is a message from your animal that she wants to feel more alive, and one of the best ways to respond to this call is through pleasurable movement.

When you get into the habit of moving every day, you'll want to make healthy food choices because you'll see the connection between what you are eating and how it makes you feel: the highest-quality foods are the ones that will give you the most energy to dance, walk, or move in any way you feel inspired. Plus, you won't feel like you're forcing yourself to be healthy because your movement will create a cascade of positivity that makes you want to honor yourself as a goddess who deserves the best care. When you let the pleasure of moving and playing lead the way, you tap into what Theresa Stevens calls "body joy."

PLEASURE PRACTICE
Where Do You Dedicate Your Time?

An interesting exercise is to take a look at how you spend your time during any typical week. Notice how much time you allow for connecting with your mind versus connecting with your body through movement, sensuality, sexuality, play, or any other form of embodiment. Give yourself permission to dedicate more time to experiencing and pleasuring your body through movements that you enjoy. Schedule it, make it a part of your day, and look forward to it. Remember, your body deserves to be treated like an equal partner to your mind, and making time for movement is one of the ways you honor her.

DANCE TO FEEL SEXY AND BEAUTIFUL

A welcome bridge from punishing exercise to pleasurable movement is dance. Dance is a sensual celebration and a potent way to reclaim your body as an instrument of delight. Dance makes embodiment fun and connects us to the greater whole of life. It is a form of movement meditation, where the mind can rest and let go of stress, while you feel beautiful in your body.

You may think dance is not a real workout, but it is actually both an aerobic and an anaerobic workout at the same time. Even when I'm feeling tired or burned out, I know that after a dance class, I'll feel more energized and connected with my body.

When you dance, you connect with yourself through movement and with the universal language of music. Joyful music inspires movement: when we are dancing to loud, rhythmic music it always feels like a party. Soft, relaxing music creates a soothing mood for the awareness-based movement practices like yoga. Aarona Pichinson is a yoga teacher who produces events called Yoga Soundscape, where a yoga class is set to live music.

She explained to me why music is so important to movement: "Music and our moods are closely related, with different types of music having different effects on our emotions. Music helps us slow down our overthinking mind and encourages us to be in our senses. Music subtly guides our movement without telling us what to do. It makes you feel that you can relax and let go a little more. Different types of music get you into different parts of the body. Some music gets you into your hips, and other music connects you with your heart. You'll feel the rhythm moving through you, like a metronomic pulse."

While I'm all for dancing alone at home, there is great pleasure to be found when dancing with others. Search out live music or dance environments where you can cut loose. Look for Five Rhythms, Ecstatic Dance, and contact improvisation jams in your area.

PLEASURE PRACTICE
Your Private Dance

Make a playlist of three songs, put them on, and move. If you are extra brave, do it in front of a mirror. And if you are extra, extra brave, do it naked in front of a mirror.

DISCOVER THE PLEASURABLE ART OF BELLY DANCE

My greatest love in the realm of dance is belly dance. I had my first taste of belly dance when I was living in India. I met an American belly dance teacher who offered me a private lesson. Even though I was practicing yoga several hours a day, a one-hour belly dance class introduced me to muscles I didn't even know I had. My abs were sore for days! Yet the movement immediately felt natural, as if she were teaching me a language I already knew.

Belly dance is the oldest form of dance for women and is designed to complement the feminine body. It originated as a ritual celebration and reenactment of the birthing process, as well as a physical preparation for creating the elasticity, mobility, strength, and connectivity necessary for an easy childbirth. Though it is called belly dance, above all, this dance gets you into your hips. Because our culture is so mind oriented, many women are disconnected from the lower parts of their bodies. The media's depiction of beauty as a boyish, anorexic-looking runway model with no boobs or hips is a stark contrast to the voluptuous full figure most women have, and it makes us ashamed of and even more disconnected from our hips, which are our greatest source of power.

In yoga, *shakti* is the word for the universal feminine energy of creation, which is stored in the lower abdominal area, the womb, and the ovaries, protected by the hips. When you have a powerful relationship with your hips and lower body, you have a direct connection to the source of feminine power. Through belly dance, we develop an awareness and appreciation for the hips and the lower part of the body, and when we do, we feel more content. Belly dance connects us with the earth.

Feeling centered in your hips makes you feel grounded and gives you a sense of security. The more you are centered in your hips, the more creative you will feel. You'll also feel healthier, more conscious, and more alive. Even if you are self-conscious, after an hour of moving your hips, your heart opens, you smile, you feel empowered, and you begin to love your body, because you feel perfect just the way you are.

The beautiful thing about going to a belly dance class is that you'll see every shape and form of body joyously welcomed in the room. My teacher, Tenley Wallace, says, "Belly dance is largely a tribal, community experience. Traditionally it has been handed from mother to daughter and conducted in the most supportive environment, in which women cheer each other on. It is an atmosphere of women adoring women. Dancing with women is an amazing opportunity to have yourself reflected back in a positive way." In the belly dance community, negativity is actively discouraged. I can't recall ever attending a class that was catty, bitchy, or competitive. In a world where isolation is a common experience and where we're constantly being pulled out of our center, belly dance brings us back to our roots. When we move our bodies rhythmically in the same space as others, something magical happens. When you dance, you feel connected to the music, to your sisters, and to yourself—and you're definitely not alone.

There are three important movements in belly dance: circles, undulations, and shimmies, all of which are signatures of pleasurable moment. Punishing approaches are often linear, like lunging or racing to a finish line. But the feminine form is based on circles: we have round hips, tummies, breasts, and wombs. Ironically, the ubiquitous quest for a flat belly overlooks the fact that the feminine body is fundamentally round. All over the world you'll find that circles and spirals are ancient symbols of the goddess. Belly dancing incorporates all of these deeper meanings into its circular movements.

Undulations show us that our bodies are composed largely of liquid and are intended to be fluid in movement. Undulations free us energetically and create a flexible and healthy spine that will support us for a lifetime. They awaken what yoga describes as *kundalini,* a serpentine energy that is stored in the lower spine and can cause profound, altered states of consciousness. Undulating also connects us with our sexuality: when we become fluid, we feel more sexual. Dara Cole, owner of Sacred Brooklyn movement studio, once told me, "When I put on certain music, I'll often see my daughter undulate on her own. Her body just does it automatically because it feels really good. I think we lose touch with that innocent expression when we're told that it's not an appropriate way to move." Shimmies shake out stagnation from your body and mind, just like a moving river keeps the water clear. The shimmy of the shoulders, of the hips, in fact of the whole body adds sensual energy to any type of dance. This type of movement also makes you feel like you are on top of the world.

Belly dancing is widely available. Because these movements are so innate to the female body, it's easy to learn and enjoy. I learned through a combination of going to classes and following instructional DVDs. No matter your shape, age, or background, belly dance can be a pleasurable experience. It's low-impact, invigorating, and tailor made for a woman's body.

PLEASURE PRACTICE
Investigate Sensual Forms of Dance

There are many other forms of dance that offer benefits similar to belly dance, including African dance, samba, hip hop, and Bollywood dance. These dance forms require that you use your whole body and, in particular, that you bend your knees when you dance. This helps you develop lower-body strength, which has the greatest effect on changing your metabolic rate.

In addition, you can find dedicated classes for sensual movement, including pole dancing or burlesque. Contrary to the stereotype, pole dancing is accessible to all body types. Dara Cole says she hears so many women tell her that at first they have a lot of apprehension, often saying, "Oh, I'm not sexy," and then fifteen minutes into the class, they're so connected to their bodies that they report, "This is the first time I've felt sexy in a long while." Dara says that pole dancing is like sex on the dance floor, and with continuous practice, you'll definitely feel sexier.

SALSA: DANCE AS PRAYER

As odd as it may sound, one of the best things that ever happened to me was being stood up by a girlfriend at a salsa club. Something came up for her at the last minute, and I ended up in a situation I would not have voluntarily put myself in, being alone in a nightclub. That night, however, I discovered I could safely and pleasurably navigate a nightclub by myself, and so I began going to salsa clubs by myself on a regular basis. I learned the basic steps of salsa in a friend's living room and then took some classes. I bought proper salsa shoes and learned the rest on the dance floor.

I was raised listening to classical music, which is characterized by complex melodies that float to the sky, in the direction of a heavenly realm. Salsa, with its wild and wanton rhythms, has an entirely different spiritual emphasis: it drums praise down into the earth. Salsa draws its roots from earth-based African spiritual traditions. The *salseros* focus on the earth because that is the source of life. Each step on the dance floor is as deliberate as each sound of the drum and is a reminder of where all life originates—Mother Earth. Salsa's movements are inherently sexual and prompt us to pay attention to our hips and the raw energies that animate our bodies.

At the base of salsa music are the drums, which weave a rhythmic web of beats that ensnare the dancer. They are designed to be hypnotic. Overlaid are the melodies that repeat like mantras, deepening the hook the music has on the psyche. In the depths of such a relaxing yet invigorating state, the whirring thoughts of the mind quiet down, and peace descends. As I dance, I feel the medicine of the music tranquilizing my mind and washing away layers of stress. Salsa makes me feel ecstatic and oh so alive.

Salsa is one of many partner dances—including tango, ballroom dance, and swing dancing—that provides a model of etiquette between men and women. It demonstrates how opposite sexes can relate in a synergistic, respectful, and sensual way. Women come to be appreciated as artistic partners rather than sexual objects. The men I've become friends with through salsa dance have been consummate gentlemen who carry this reverent attitude toward women off the dance floor.

Within salsa, there are many other rituals going on, outside of the dance itself. These include the practice of asking someone to dance, the subsequent accepting or declining of the invitation, the subtle signaling that one wants to be asked to dance, saying goodbye at the end, and switching partners. It amazes me how I can dance intimately in the arms of a stranger for five minutes and then be passed along to another and another, all in complete safety.

The dance floor provides an ideal environment for cultivating honest communication. This is perfectly portrayed in the movie *Take the Lead*. Antonio Banderas's character, Pierre Dulaine, volunteers to teach Latin and ballroom dancing in New York City schools. When the relevance of his work is challenged by a narrow-minded teacher, who threatens the future of his class, he explains the deeper benefits: "If your sixteen-year-old daughter allows me to lead, she is trusting me, but more than that, she is trusting herself. And if she is strong, secure, and trusts herself, then how likely is she to let some idiot knock her up? And if your son can learn to touch women with respect, how will he treat women throughout his life? I teach dance, and with it a set of rules that will teach your children about trust, teamwork, and dignity."

I admire the importance Latin culture gives to dance. It delights me that Latin culture deems dance a necessary ingredient for the fullest expression of both femininity and masculinity. In salsa, it appears that the man is leading, but energetically both the man and the woman create the dance. As Dulaine went on to say in the film, "In salsa, the man leads, or rather he proposes the step. It is the woman's choice to follow." Partner dance relies on mastering nonverbal communication. As you learn to do it with your dance partner, you also learn to do it with your animal.

I recommend you take salsa classes, and as soon as you have the courage, attend dance socials and dance clubs as well. Maybe you think you have two left feet and couldn't possibly learn to salsa dance, but rest assured that in classes, the steps are taught in bite-sized chunks. If you can walk, you can dance. All it takes is showing up.

SALUTE YOUR HIGHER SELF WITH YOGA

The form of movement that first changed my life and my body was yoga. I can recommend this practice to every woman because of the diversity it offers. There is a flavor for everyone. Dating back thousands of years to ancient India, yoga has always been a fusion of spirituality and physicality, and for that reason, it perfectly captures the principles of pleasurable movement. It's not just about how you move but also about how you think and feel. Although today in the West, yoga is generally associated with physical postures, in its entirety, yoga is a philosophy for living, based on the principle of nonviolence, including nonviolence to one's self. If you are looking to get away from the punishing exercise paradigm, yoga is a great place to start, and it is now widely available.

The foundation of yoga is awareness—in particular, awareness of your breath. Because your breath is the most powerful tool to move you out of the stress response and into the weight loss–promoting relaxation response, yoga is a most effective way to establish the metabolism for lasting weight loss. The ability to relax into intensity that you learn on the yoga mat can be applied to any situation in life where you need to deal with intensity.

The physical practice of yoga is the practice of *asanas,* or poses, which help you build strength, flexibility and balance, and release stress and tension from the body. Each asana offers its own specific therapeutic benefits. The styles of yoga vary immensely, and there are new styles being pioneered all the time. For example, you can choose a challenging and fast-paced style like vinyasa yoga, a more moderate practice like anusara yoga, or a relaxing and slow-paced form like restorative yoga. All of the styles are preparation for the practice of sitting meditation.

Although yoga is popular among the young, fit, and flexible, don't let that discourage you from starting. There are gentle beginner classes that can accommodate you at your present shape. If you go to a class and feel uncomfortable, try another. Restorative yoga is a particularly good place to start if you have been inactive because it will help you gently open your joints. Restorative yoga includes the use of props to put your body into positions where you can reach a state of total comfort, tranquility, and nonexertion. The goal of restorative yoga is to relax the nervous system as deeply as possible so that restoration and healing, including weight loss, can occur. Restorative yoga teaches us that movement doesn't have to be intense to be effective in altering your metabolism.

Yoga is an introspective experience where you are encouraged to focus your attention on your own practice instead of looking around the room and comparing yourself to others. Consequently, the only person paying attention to you is the instructor, so you don't need to feel self-conscious as you learn to master the poses. Yoga centers are often community hubs and offer a great place to meet new friends. The way to greet someone in yoga is to put your hands together in a prayer position in front of your heart and say, "Namaste," which means "My higher self salutes your higher self."

THE FASTEST WAY TO LOOK TEN POUNDS LIGHTER

I had been working with my client Roberta for over a year. She had already lost forty pounds in a pleasurable, enlivening way and was aiming to lose another twenty. One day she walked into my office looking remarkably different. "You look like you have lost ten pounds since I saw you last week," I said.

It turns out that Roberta didn't lose weight overnight. Instead, she had learned how to improve her posture, which changed her appearance entirely. Roberta had met with posture expert Gina Schatz, who taught her how to engage her intrinsic muscles. These are not the core muscles you use doing sit-ups, but ones you can engage whether you're at your desk, walking, or just moving around the house. Roberta learned that anyone can have a toned body, even if you're not lifting weights, as long as you are activating your intrinsic muscles.

Most women are familiar with the phasic muscles—quadriceps, biceps, triceps, and hamstrings. However, what gives dancers their grace and beauty, which is what all women want, is that their movement is always about lifting up, which requires activating the finer, intrinsic muscles that lie along our bones. You have intrinsic muscles in your hands and feet and along your back. These muscles provide stability to every move you make, and when activated mindfully, they can improve both posture and balance.

PLEASURE PRACTICE
How to Have Perfect Posture

The basic rule of thumb for good posture, as taught by Gina Schatz, is to create a straight line up and down your body. Position your ears above your shoulders by drawing your ears (or your ponytail) directly behind you without tilting your chin back, as opposed to leaning your head forward (as most people do most of the time). Position your shoulder blades as flat as possible on your back without sticking your chest out. Position your ribs directly over your hips, as opposed to jutting them out too far forward or slouching too far back. Position your hips over your knees, as opposed to thrusting them forward or tilting them back in a sway back. And lastly, position your knees over your ankles, as opposed to hyperextending or locking them. When you correctly align your bones, you will feel as poised as a queen. Standing in that regal posture, you will also feel invincible.

THE ANCIENT ART OF SQUATTING
In addition to circles, undulations, and shimmies, the fourth quintessential feminine movement is squatting. Visit India and you will see people squatting everywhere. They squat while cooking, eating, waiting for the bus, and chatting with friends. Privately, women in India squat while giving birth and going to the bathroom. But our culture doesn't value squatting. We prefer to sit on chairs and give birth lying on our backs. Our hips are

on lockdown. We don't know how to use that part of the body, and we pay the price with rampant back pain and inflexible hips.

Squatting is a way to give some love to your hips, and it has innumerable benefits. It develops elasticity in your hips, knees, and ankles; aids digestion; engages your pelvic floor; develops balance; lengthens the spine; and most important, is grounding. It brings your energy down to your feminine power center. If you don't yet have that range of motion, squatting is going to feel like a lot of work for you, but as you develop flexibility in your hips, squatting will become a comfortable position.

You can squat anywhere, any time. To start squatting and developing your flexibility, you may want to rest your heels on a folded blanket so that it is more comfortable. I taught my friend Annie the power of squatting, and she has told me that when she's emotionally triggered or overwhelmed, she will squat on the floor to ground and center herself. Tenley Wallace told me she makes it a point to squat for a few minutes before leaving the house. When I squat, I feel like a bird, perched and ready to fly at a moment's notice, and deeply connected with my animal nature and her wisdom.

DEVELOPING MUSCLE SUPPORTS PLEASURABLE WEIGHT LOSS

Fitness expert Andréa Albright believes that the biggest mistake women make while trying to transform their bodies is doing a thousand sit-ups or hours of cardio when they really need to be building muscle. Just as relaxation puts you in a beneficial metabolic state, developing your muscles puts you in a beneficial physiological state. The more muscle you have, the more efficient you become at metabolizing food. You'll also have more energy to do the things you love. When you build muscle, you get leaner and tighter, and your clothes start to get looser. The number on the scale may be deceiving when you're building muscle because muscle is denser and more compact than body fat, so the scale may show your weight going up, even though you are getting smaller. Yet another reason to throw away the scale!

The best place for women to build muscle is in the lower body—your thighs and your butt—which are your largest muscle groups. Simply activating those targeted muscles increases metabolism, which affects the way you look overall, including your arms and your belly. Women who have strong muscles in their lower bodies frequently have great posture and body awareness, and also look younger.

Many fitness experts say that the most effective way to build muscle and burn abdominal fat is through interval training, where you repetitively start and stop movement in short intervals. Most people associate interval training with movements that are designed solely to make your muscles burn, like push-ups. These are also the exercises most women have a hard time committing to because they find them tedious and boring. However, interval training doesn't have to be defined by gym activities. *Interval training* is simply a modern term that describes an ancient way of moving, in short bursts in which you go fast and then slow, which is how all animals move. You'll be happy to hear that you can get the same benefits of interval training by shaking your butt on the dance floor! Playing basketball, running around the park chasing a Frisbee, and other activities that have quick starts and stops also work. While the punishing paradigm would insist that you have to go to the gym and work at your maximum intensity many days a week to build muscle and burn fat, that's simply not the case. If you enjoy resistance exercises that use your own body weight, like push-ups, planks, or inversions, feel free to include them in your movement practice. But if they don't float your boat, try something else. I've seen women transform their bodies through dance alone.

DRESS THE PART FOR PLEASURABLE MOVEMENT

Pleasurable movement is simply more fun when you have the right outfit. It's easier to love and appreciate yourself when you're wearing something you feel great in. A quality pair of yoga or dance pants can make you feel amazing. Don't assume that just because you are going to get sweaty you should wear baggy, old clothes. If you do, you'll miss out on the opportunity to enjoy wearing clothes that move and flow, in colors you like. Don't wait until you lose weight to reward yourself with clothing that will make the process more pleasurable.

The act of moving your body every day has a dramatic effect on your stress levels and your sense of personal power and pride. Any daily commitment to pleasurable movement is going to help you lose weight, while you honor your animal by giving her the best care. Some of the modalities we've discussed take time and practice to master, but they will get easier. The secret is doing it consistently by making it part of your lifestyle. Speak encouragingly to your animal with words like, "You're doing great," and you will motivate yourself to keep going. When you are done, give yourself a pat on the back for taking care of your animal and for honoring your commitment to make movement a part of your life.

The world will be saved by the Western woman.

DALAI LAMA

11 From Envy to Appreciation

WOMAN, CONGRATULATIONS for making it to here! You've been on an epic journey to get to know your female animal with fresh eyes. You've learned to love her form and love yourself like never before. You've learned to reinvent your ecology. You've started to feel safe looking and feeling as sexy as you want. You're eating with intention, cooking with delight, and moving with pleasure. Still, there's one last magical ingredient that holds this pleasurable approach to weight loss together and makes it sustainable. Nothing in nature exists in isolation. Each of us is a part of the whole, and in order to succeed, we need one another. That's the last secret to pleasurable weight loss: we can't do it alone. Your community provides the sense of belonging, inspiration, and support you need to sustain change in your life and, therefore, your body. Embrace the sisterhood, the universal kinship of all women.

When I ended my struggle with food and weight more than ten years ago, I thought I'd feel on top of the world. I had a thriving business, I was dating and having great sex, I was part of a creative scene in New York City and attending avant-garde parties with fascinating people, but I still felt like something was missing in my life. By this time, I was becoming well known locally as a health coach. My photograph was in magazines, and I would often be stopped at the local health food restaurant—"Are you Jena?" Anyone would have presumed I had tons of friends, but the truth was, I felt lonely and isolated. I knew a lot of people but allowed only a few into the recesses of my heart. I concealed my fears and insecurities under a social mask. I was also emotionally guarded with the few girlfriends I did have, only exposing the parts of me that I thought would appeal to them and covering up the darker parts I thought might repel them. I focused most of my attention on my achievements and kept myself busy. Conveniently, I didn't have time for the friends I didn't have.

Over time my loneliness intensified. It became apparent that having the body of my dreams and a successful career wasn't enough to make me happy, and maintaining the charade of having it all was making me miserable. Something had to change because it felt meaningless to go on living in such emotional isolation. I remember one year when my birthday rolled around I wanted to throw myself a birthday party with women, but I couldn't figure out who to invite. I knew many women but privately held judgments and criticisms about each one. One wasn't ambitious enough, another wasn't confident enough, one wasn't spiritual enough, another was too corporate, this one was too hippy, this one had a boyfriend I thought was a loser. I used my judgments to rationalize walls of separation between the other women and me, and I feared being judged in the same way by them.

At the same time I was learning about the concept of accountability and the suffering obligations of love. I started to become aware that wherever I went in life, I was accustomed to writing myself the script of a victim, constantly feeling let down and disappointed by one thing or another, and this was playing out in my friendships with women. I also saw how I was living out a suffering obligation of love to my mother to be lonely and isolated the way she was. As these realizations sank in, I understood that I was the cause of my own loneliness and that in reality there was a sisterhood I could engage with right at my fingertips—a world of women available to connect with me if only I would take the initiative.

Determined to change my inner and outer ecologies, I began to proactively participate in workshops and group programs so that I could connect with women in an authentic way. I was ready to create the meaningful relationships my soul was hungry for. Instead of blaming other women, I became the one who would initiate getting together for one-on-one lunches, creating a safe and comfortable setting for emotional intimacy to deepen. Most important, I learned to expose my vulnerability: I made it a point to share the things I used to hide. I let others see where I didn't have it all together. I also shared the triumphs and victories that previously I would have held private. I began to realize that the women around me wanted to be close to all of me, not just my public image. My judgments against these women had been my devices for maintaining distance from them, but they were actually amazing beings with so much to offer in friendship.

As I did this, an amazing thing happened. One day I felt a shift occur. It was as if the fabric of reality changed in an instant. One moment I felt alone, as if I was fending for myself in a threatening world, and the next, I felt intimately connected, as if I was part of a web of women with whom I could give and receive. Right then I knew that I belonged to a community, a sisterhood.

The more I made female friendship a non-negotiable priority in my life and embraced the principle of transparency, the happier I became. After years of doing this, I now find myself thoroughly enmeshed in a community of women I love deeply, who love me, support me, lean on me, and are with me. They witness me as I move through the ups and downs of life, and I witness them. I think of these women as my sisters, my tribeswomen, and united with their powerful and diverse feminine energy, I feel there is nothing life can throw at me that I cannot make it through.

When you feel supported by your sisters, you don't have to turn to food for comfort, no matter how intense the day or the phase of your life is. You have other avenues for processing your emotions. You feel held by the unconditional love of women who know your light and your darkness and appreciate you for your totality. Without sisterhood, the pain of loneliness is so intense and stressful, it sabotages everything else. But when you can completely relax and let down your guard with your close friends, you experience the relaxation that is at the heart of sustainable weight loss.

This is the support system that I want you to have as you devote yourself to the path of pleasurable weight loss. As you embrace living with pleasure, commit yourself to the well-being of your female animal, and reap the benefits of a renewed and healed relationship with food, I want you to experience the refreshing and loving support of a sisterhood with every fumbling, elegant, or daring step you take.

Like pleasure, sisterhood is an ancient need; without it, our feminine souls wither and our animals suffer. The more quality connections we experience in our lives, the happier we feel. Women have such a biological need for social bonding that our bodies literally malfunction without it. Blood pressure increases, altering our psychology, making us depressed and anxious. Being separate from other women is simply not what nature intended. Since the cave days, we have continued to evolve living together. Evolutionary psychology observes that the most distinctive traits of our species are the pleasure it gives us to come together to collaborate and how good we are at it. Women have historically spent our days together, watching children, gathering and preparing food, and tending to home and hearth. "No matter what you were feeling, even if you wanted to isolate yourself, you would be very seen, felt, celebrated, and held by your sisters," says personal coach and sisterhood advocate Nisha Moodley. This puts into perspective our current predicament of feeling disconnected from sisterhood as a relatively modern phenomenon. Prior to the pervasive lifestyle of the single-family home, we all lived in extended family configurations, so there was no way to avoid sisterhood.

Today we experience an unprecedented separation among women. Just as our culture has not appreciated and fostered the feminine values of collaboration and community, we have not been conditioned to appreciate the importance, depth, and legacy of sisterhood. "We've been taught to appear successful at all costs, putting our best face forward and striving to look perfectly put together to show the world how perfect things are at home, regardless of how we actually feel," says Nisha Moodley. "We've felt discouraged from sharing our feelings about our insecurities or problems and consequently learned to soothe ourselves with food."

However, when we return to a sisterhood and feel comfortable revealing our true selves, we can have healthy emotional lives. With the unconditional love of sisterhood, we can express our fear, anger, pain, jealousy, and other emotions so that they move through us like a wave, instead of being stagnant and becoming toxic. And when we can fully experience our emotional range without reservation, we can finally be one with our animals. With a sisterhood to listen to us, we can also support and listen to our animals.

MOVING PAST COMPARISON DESPAIR

In contrast to the earth-based feminine value that recognizes we belong to the abundance of nature and so there is always enough, our modern-day culture, based on masculine values, teaches us that competition is the only way to get ahead. We have been indoctrinated to think that there's a limited amount of resources (men, sex, money, career success, etc.) and that when other women succeed, there is less for the rest of us. It's the same meme we've explored throughout the book: the feeling of not having enough and not being enough. The logical side effect of scarcity thinking is that we feel envious of other women. If you are threatened by women who have the body and the looks you desire and it makes you spiteful, it's a sign that you need to shift your perspective from a scarcity mentality to an abundance mentality.

How you relate with other women is not a footnote to your relationship with your weight. When I was struggling with food and my weight, envy was a familiar emotion. I couldn't help but resent the women who had the bodies I wanted. I would gaze at them and try to conceal that I was looking—my heart wincing. I condemned my body, judging it inferior to their beauty, which created a chronic low-level stress that held me back from having the body I wanted for years.

We've been conditioned to compete with other women, which manifests as our harsh examination of women's bodies. This is the same way we've been conditioned to treat our animals, with scrutiny, judgment, comparison, and objectification. We spend vast amounts of mental energy analyzing and comparing ourselves in detail to other women, as we strive to establish our superiority but more often find our inferiority. *Comparison despair* is a term coined by personal finance expert Alexis Neely to describe the despair that arises from comparing ourselves to others. The source of comparison despair is our repressed desires, which can spill out in the form of envy. The secret to both overcoming envy and to getting what we desire is to convert comparison despair into deep appreciation.

When you begin to appreciate beautiful and slim women instead of envying them, you see them in a positive light. The truth is, every woman in every moment is trying to be her best self, to embody her unique expression of the divine feminine. Each time you see a woman walk by you, no matter what she looks like, imagine she is presenting her own version of what it means to be a woman. Once you can view this as a performance of womanhood, instead of feeling jealous or competitive, you can let a pleasurable flush of appreciation wash over you so that you can be genuinely happy for her, as well as inspired and motivated to explore what she demonstrates is possible for you. Sisterhood means giving a leg up to any woman who is reaching for something better for herself.

Alexis told me her story: "I used to have a lot of envy, and it kept me from forming relationships with women. When I discovered that envy actually points us toward what we want, then my whole attitude shifted. I let my envy draw me to appreciate women, to lift them up, praise them publicly, acknowledge their beauty, their grace, their sexiness, their smartness, their business savvy, or whatever it was that I was most envying. Instead of trying to push away, ignore, hide, or shrink the envy, I did the exact opposite and glorified it. This started moving me toward what I wanted and has ultimately led me to have what I wanted." When you are in appreciation and celebration of a woman, you see beyond her size into the magnificence of the woman she is inside, and it helps you do the same for yourself. In doing so, you break free from the toxic interpretation of envy and instead author an existence focused on pleasure.

PLEASURE PRACTICE
Convert Envy to Praise

If you find yourself caught in comparison despair and are waiting for it to go away when you lose weight, I want you to be free of its clutches right now by using this practice to remove a layer of chronic stress and provide you with a powerful tool for feeling more connected with other women. It will also help you to identify what you want and move toward having it. It's natural to feel envious, but how you react to it is up to you. When you see a woman whose body (or anything else) you envy, make a practice of internally praising that woman for those attributes or accomplishments. Recognize that what she has is a positive sign that what you desire is possible for you, too.

THE SECRET SAUCE OF SISTERHOOD

I believe that sisterhood is the secret sauce to sustainable weight loss. After reinventing my relationship to sisterhood, I now have unprecedented pleasure and much less stress in my life. I belong to a tribe of women who constantly lift one another up. I take so much pleasure in the women around me. The sweetness of a good conversation will always be more satisfying than a bowl of ice cream, and in the face of an opportunity to meaningfully connect with other women, sugar cravings fizzle. Loving our sisters helps us love ourselves, and loving and accepting their bodies as beautiful dissolves the shame we feel about our own.

Sisterhood provides a pleasure that is incomparable to any other. As embodiment expert Michaela Boehm says, "The feminine heart needs to be seen, felt, met, and understood. It's really important that women are seen by each other." That's why I want you, as the author of your life, to be proactively immersing yourself in the company of other women. To feel your best as a woman, you need to find women who can reflect your beauty back to you because they are connected to their own beauty. They can illuminate the path and show you the way. We are mirroring creatures. Simply being in a room with other women will teach you something new. And that's particularly true for your relationship with your body. When you are in the presence of women who are experiencing pleasure in their body, eating nourishing foods, dressing with style, and living true to their feminine heart, you will be affected. Being with a woman who clearly loves her animal is instructional without her ever saying a word.

When you have good women friends supporting you, you can take risks to explore new ideas and test the edges of your pleasure threshold. For example, the positive encouragement of your girlfriends may inspire you to wear a sexy outfit that, left to your own devices, you may not have worn. You might start going to movement classes or make healthier choices with food. Knowing how to have solid, intimate, caring relationships with women will make you feel safe and more confident. Amber Lupton, coauthor of *Give Peace a Deadline,* says, "When you are not afraid to talk to another woman, say hello, look her in the eye to make yourself known, then you'll feel safer wherever you go. You will always feel supported."

CREATING SISTERHOOD

The next step is to find a pleasure-positive community of sisters that supports your new lifestyle choices. Instead of waiting and hoping your social circle will miraculously transform, become the instigator who makes it happen. Most women are yearning for more pleasure, and it sometimes only takes one woman in the social group to say, "Hey, why don't we meet at my house, dress up and go out, hang out, drink tea, dance, or give each other foot massages?"

Invite a few girlfriends over, put music on, dance, and delight in your senses. Dress up in the zany outfits you don't wear in public. Organize a day trip to a Korean spa, where all the women are naked, from grandmothers to young girls, and everyone scrubs each other clean. In doing so, you situate yourself in a safe ecology in which to feel sensual and experience new pleasures. When we embrace the values of pleasure and sisterhood, we relish the fact that it is available to everyone. This democratic nature of pleasure means that the more people are enjoying themselves, the more pleasurable it is. This principle can help you create a social scene that is nourishing and pleasurable for all.

When you want to make any transformation, there is no more powerful way to support this than by interacting and socializing with other people who already have what you want or are on their way to having it. If women want to develop new friendships, do what Nisha Moodley calls "friend dating." By surrounding yourself with women who share your goals and values, possess a pleasure-positive attitude, and wholeheartedly believe in what's possible for you, you'll be able to attain your desires as if by osmosis. This is the feminine strategy of designing your ideal ecology in action.

My client Debbie was a regular attendee at my Pleasure Camps. She says that her life was transformed by embracing sisterhood. "Before I met you, I didn't realize that sisterhood was the magic missing in my life. By embracing sisterhood, I now bathe in the love of other women. I have always cheered others on, yet I didn't permit others to do the same for me. I was afraid of someone seeing 'behind the curtain.' Allowing women to cheer me on has helped me let go of so much of the emotional weight, which had been dragging me down and keeping me in the vicious cycle of bad body image in which I compared myself to others, triggering me to make poor food choices that gave me no satisfaction.

"I've now come to see every woman as my sister, someone to support, assist, guide, and love. I now know that every woman is beautiful in her own unique way. I celebrate individuality and the coming together to engage, play, and create. Being in a loving community of sisters with no agenda but to heal from within and with one another, I began to realize that my body is an expression of my soul and that when my soul is truly happy, my body expresses that joy, too. I have reconnected with my heart's desires, like a baby who cries when she's hungry and pushes away the bottle when she is not.

"Without the loving connection of sisterhood I would not feel this comfortable in my body or this confident living a pleasurable lifestyle. I now actually feel pretty, have lost 20 pounds, have toned my body, and am even excited to wear a bikini this summer! When I ask myself, 'Which came first, reconnection with myself or connecting with others?' the answer is they came at the very same time."

By demonstrating the principles of pleasurable living and by creating traditions and practices within your social group, you can become what I call a "culture maker." For example, I have helped seed a pleasure-positive attitude in my community so that now it is the norm of my social group. Through the conversations you have with other women, the events you host, and the ideas you share, you, too, can seed a subculture in which all of your sisters embrace pleasure, just as you have.

PLEASURE PRACTICE
Create a Sister Circle

The Goddess Artemis is the goddess of female communities, our wild animal nature, and our intuition. She is a reminder that women have been gathering in groups or circles throughout our evolution. There's no better way to cultivate sisterhood than by creating an intentional sister circle, where women can get together to share and bond. A sister circle can be a weekly or monthly affair, in person or by phone. For example, I am part of a sister circle, and we call ourselves the Mistress Mind (as opposed to a mastermind). Eight girlfriends meet by phone for an hour a week. We can bring anything to the call, and we support one another in every way.

It's easy to lead a sister circle because there is no required formula. The basic guideline is to create a sacred space and give each woman time to share without being interrupted. A powerful practice is to invite the women in your sister circle to be your witnesses, as you declare your intentions. This way, you are giving others the opportunity to help you be accountable for attaining your desires. As you give each other space to share honestly, you'll discover how your friends are going through similar experiences. It's uplifting, empowering, and soothing to know that we are not alone.

THE PLEASURE OF DEEP RELATIONSHIPS
One of the secrets of nourishing female friendships is transparency: revealing, sharing your hidden truths, and the willingness to be authentic and vulnerable. The truth is, a lot of women want

friends, but not everyone is emotionally and spiritually ready for the kind of deep, honest, soulful connection I am talking about. Women tell me all the time, "I can't really share with my friends what's in my heart. They would never understand." If you don't feel comfortable sharing the truth of your emotional life with your closest friends, you risk burying your emotions by overeating. While it's easy to maintain shallow friendships, what's really going to feed your soul are the deeper relationships, where you feel completely comfortable sharing your most private thoughts and feelings. When you create safe relationships where you can express your deepest emotions, you won't have to run to the fridge when you are distressed. Your friends will be there for you.

Courageously stretch yourself to go beneath the surface in your conversations, delving deeper so that you can get to know your friends on a meaningful level. When we commiserate around life's annoyances as a way of creating intimacy, it doesn't feel nourishing. Nisha says, "Even if you feel the inclination to isolate yourself or talk about the weather because it feels easy, it is not nourishing to your feminine soul." Nisha suggests that friends focus on the deeper questions and the bigger celebrations: "We all have questions that we don't have answers to and things we are excited to share." Ask women what they love doing when they are not working, what is important to them, and what projects they are excited about. If you feel shy or nervous or scared to say something for fear of sounding weird, then definitely say it, because it is an authentic expression of what you are currently feeling. Remember, deep honest relationships forge true intimacy. Cultivate relationships with women where you can talk about everything, knowing that they can hold your confidence, and you will hold theirs.

One way to be capable of bringing your deep, honest, grounded self to any relationship is to first deeply connect with the ultimate feminine energy, Mother Earth, by spending time in nature. Whether it is a forest, a park, a sunset viewing, or a moon gazing, when you are more connected to the earth, it's going to help you connect to women on a deeper level. When you feel held and loved and at one with nature, you have a certain energy that is both grounded and sparkly that other women will pick up on, and they will gravitate toward you.

PLEASURE PRACTICE
Who Are Your Allies?

Because there are millions of women in the world and you want to find your women, your tribe, your gang, your inner circle, you want to develop the ability to filter for the women who are going to hold strong intentions for you and raise you up. Make a list of the women and men you know who would be a positive support to your commitment to pleasure. Then write a second list of the areas where you need and want more support and encouragement for bringing pleasure into your life. How can you strengthen the relationships with your existing allies and cast your net to meet more allies?

TIME *TO BE* INSTEAD OF TO DO

We live in a fast-paced world, and as modern women, we are constantly doing something, if not many things, at once. One of the reasons busy women become isolated and are susceptible to weight gain is that we don't perceive spending time with other women as productive. Yet ironically, that is exactly what we need—a break from being productive! While there's a great joy in accomplishing your goals and being productive with other women, if you are already extremely busy, making a point to do more with other women will not nourish you. Instead of making yourself even busier doing more together, make a point to connect with your sisters through pleasurable activities that allow you simply to be in each other's company. These can include going to yoga, dancing together, and doing things that connect you to the earth, like taking a hike or cooking together. Embodiment expert Ariel White says, "Things that are sensual, things that are 'mindless' in a good way, like singing and dancing, that take you out of your mind and into your body will feel really nourishing to share with your female friends. If you go straight from do-do-doing to getting a pedicure with your friend where you are still texting on your phone, it won't give you the nourishing kind of sister connection that you're really craving."

So if you're thinking, "I hang out with my girlfriends all the time," it's important to look at quality versus quantity. Even one hour a week spent in a high-quality activity, like dancing or sharing deeply, where you are completely present to each other, can be profoundly satisfying to you and your animal.

THE POWER OF PLAY

Now that you've come to see the importance of sisterhood and you've sought out the friendship of great women, what are you going to do together? You would think that my answer would be to seek pleasure, but there's a specific type of pleasure that is the secret that gives sisterhood its full pizazz—play! Pleasure and play are cousins. Neither is a luxury, a distraction, or an indulgence. Play is one of the few universal traits that all animals share, making it a critical ingredient for a satisfied life. When you play, you are deeply connected to your animal, which is the state of being where losing weight is naturally pleasurable.

The nature of play is to make us feel more alive, creative, and connected to the full spectrum of our emotional range. Play brings you into the present moment and makes you less self-conscious. When you play, you take a break from the mundane and stressful activities of life, and through sensing what feels good from moment to moment, your animal has a chance to relax. Like eating, play gives you an opportunity to pay attention to what gives your animal delight. So often fulfilling our daily responsibilities can box us into specific predictable ways of being, and play brings the spice of life back into the daily mix. Play requires improvisation and cultivates the ability to make things up as you go. Play and curiosity go hand in hand; without play there is no evolution. That's why cutting-edge companies like Google pay their employees to play: it stimulates innovation. All of these aspects of play are directly related to the secrets of pleasurable weight loss.

Your struggle with weight and food may be an indicator of a play deficiency. When play is absent, seriousness takes over, and we become contracted, dry, sad versions of ourselves. As adults we are prone to take ourselves too seriously, to the great detriment of our health and well-being. In the absence of the primal nourishment of play, we are also vulnerable to cravings for sugar or alcohol, in an attempt to relieve the stress caused by the lack of play and ease in your life. If satisfying play is not present in your life, it's a telltale sign that you are creating a martyr role for yourself, taking pride in your personal sacrifices of trivialities like play and pleasure.

No matter how you feel about your body, you can play with your sisters right now. All you need is the willingness to be present and openhearted. Embodiment expert Amy Dawn Verebay encourages us to "approach play with wonder and a beginner's mind, letting go your preconceived notions of what your body can or can't do." When you have built up a lifetime of invulnerability, embracing the childlike state of play may make you feel exposed, but as soon as you are willing to give it a go, you will find your animal is always waiting and wanting to play.

PLEASURE PRACTICE
How Do You Like to Play?

Visualize your inner seven-year-old. Ask her, "How do you most like to play?" She might suggest blowing bubbles, playing dress up, talking with fairies, making music, cooking, or running outside. Then ask your adult animal how she would most like to play. Her answer might be playful lovemaking, rolling in the grass in the park, swimming in the ocean, dancing, or singing. Schedule nonstructured time into your day so that you can play for at least ten minutes every day. Dedicate this time to fun, freedom, and getting into a relaxing flow. Make a list of friends whose company inspires you to play, and make it a point to spend time with these women.

THE HEALING POWERS OF SONG

Cultural anthropologist Angeles Arrien described how the ancient wisdom of many shamanic societies attributed healing powers to song: "If you came to a medicine person complaining of being disheartened, dispirited, or depressed, they would ask, When did you stop singing?" Like dancing, looking for the beauty in life, and authoring your own story, singing is one of the secrets of pleasurable weight loss. It is a primordial and universal activity that women of every culture take pleasure in. Sadly, in our culture, singing is left to professionals and children, while the rest of us miss out.

I was once on a road trip with four of my closest girlfriends, and asked each of them, "Do you like singing?" The first woman answered, "I'm not good at it." The second woman said, "I don't like the way my voice sounds." The remaining two had equally self-critical responses. What they didn't realize was that they weren't answering the question directly. They were focused on judging their ability to sing, not on whether it gave them pleasure. In that moment, my girlfriends and I recognized that we had been focusing on criticism rather than enjoyment, and we became committed to not letting perfectionism stand in the way of the playful pleasure of song.

I want you to dust off your vocal cords and reclaim your birthright to this natural, free, and playful weight loss secret. When you are singing and you bring your full attention to the sound that you are creating, you are pulled away from any thought-loop that you may be caught in. For example, if you are stuck in anxiety-producing envy, you can change your state by singing. Think of singing as "mind altering" because it breaks you out of your repetitive thoughts and refocuses your attention on the present moment, which is where healing and pleasurable weight loss occur.

Like yoga, singing engages your breath, clears your mind, and connects you with the feeling of aliveness. When you sing and the resonance of the sound fills your body, it is an exquisite sensual feeling. You feel beautiful, powerful, and free. You feel connected to the depths of your being and, of course, to your animal. Singing will inspire you and will encourage you to express emotions you may otherwise be repressing. Plus, you can't be eating while you're singing. In a moment of anxiety, imagine if you started singing instead of heading toward the fridge or pantry. What if you could express, instead of repress, through song the feeling that is triggering you to overeat? Losing weight may have less to do with eating and exercising and more to do with singing more and worrying less.

PLEASURE PRACTICE
Sing with Your Animal and Your Sisters

Sing with your animal. Serenade her for the sheer delight of it and for the emotional expression it gives you. Sing in the shower, sing along to music, sing with friends, and sing while you cook. Belt out a song at the top of your lungs. Let go, cut loose! Usually our voices tend to be restrained, so any time you can let your voice be uninhibited it is a triumph. Take a simple song, which could be in any language, and teach it to your girlfriends. Then sing it together several times, letting your mind relax. Feel the power of sound and music playfully and deeply connect you with other women.

Sisterhood is the glue that holds pleasurable weight loss together. Just as there are a wide variety of pleasures for you to savor, there's a whole world of women who would be thrilled to be your friend, companion, and sister on your journey. The pursuit of pleasure, no matter the route, is a universal motivator. Open your heart and mind to the women around you. United with each other and with your female animals, there's nothing you can't accomplish.

There came a time when the risk to remain tight in the bud was more painful than the risk it took to blossom.

ANAIS NIN

epilogue The Path to Pleasure Is Sacred

MY FIRST EXPOSURE to the idea that pleasure was beneficial was when I was nineteen years old. I'd stumbled upon a book about earth-based religion written by Starhawk. In black and white, she spelled it out, "All pleasure, harm it none, is in honor of the divine." The idea sent a shock through my system. I'd never heard anything remotely like this, yet the words instantly resonated as true. Pleasure is not shameful, not even neutral; it is sacred. The act of consciously receiving pleasure connects our awareness to the very pulse of life through the senses, and in doing so, honors the divine. What better way to honor the sacred than by thoroughly enjoying our existence?

"All pleasure, harm it none," is the directive to seek pleasure without harming yourself, your animal, or anyone else, thereby satisfying the conditions for true pleasure. Pleasure shows us that the sacred is present here and now, imminent in our experience, and not something that awaits us after death or enlightenment.

The experience of pleasure doesn't have to feel like something is happening, but it does feel like nothing is missing. At some point, everyone asks the question, What is the meaning of life? My answer is pleasure. Having pleasure in life and having meaning in life are one and the same. Pleasure teaches that life itself wants to be savored, relished, and appreciated. Whenever I ask people what gives their lives meaning and why, their final responses always boil down to, "It makes me feel good," showing that whatever brings pleasure gives life meaning.

BECOME A PLEASURE ACTIVIST

You now have at your disposal all the secrets to pleasurable weight loss. You might already be experiencing a shift in how you look and feel. You might feel lighter in spirit or have set your sights on new delights that you want to incorporate into your life. Now you know that you are part of something bigger than yourself—your sisterhood—and the recognition that you are not alone will make it much easier to continue the journey.

I hope that you take pleasure in all that life offers and see food as a source of nourishment and joy, not a punishment or source of pain. The more you believe in your ability to succeed, the more likely it is you will. Serious science supports this: studies show that simply believing we can make a positive change in our lives increases our chance of success. To succeed at pleasurable weight loss, embrace the fundamental belief that you and your animal are capable of change. You are no longer a woman overcome by her struggles with weight and self-image. You are a catalyst who is changing the world.

Living in your pleasure will enhance all areas of your life that go far beyond weight loss. When you look around, you'll see women of all shapes and sizes who are not living their lives ignited by pleasure—you'll see it on their faces. Now that you know that trusting your animal and trusting pleasure is the spark they are missing, I want you to become a pleasure activist who awakens women to a pleasure-positive mind-set and supports them on their own journeys. In your own way, invite your sisters into the pleasure movement. Share what you've learned so that they, too, can intimately connect to their female animals. In turn, you will become their inspiration for living a pleasure-filled existence, so that they, too, can experience how rewarding and extraordinary this philosophy can be.

Remember: you don't have to be the martyr who ensures everyone else's pleasure, while receiving none herself. The secret is to design a lifestyle and a community where pleasure flows naturally to and from you, supporting you, enlivening you, and nurturing you to make the best possible choices for yourself and your animal. And as you go through life and come across women who are clearly trusting the infallible wisdom of their bodies and living in their pleasure, make a point to acknowledge them and let them know that you belong together in the same sisterhood. Bask in their radiant glory, and shower them with your appreciation. They know, as you now do, that a woman's pleasure is sacred.

Acknowledgments

SOMETIMES IN LIFE you come across someone whose belief in you is so great that it transforms your own opinion of yourself and what you believe you are capable of. In the realm of being an author, Michael Ellsberg was that person to me. In our early conversations, he encouraged me to envision myself as an author. He then mentored me with sage advice, and held my hand, never allowing me to give up on my dream, all the way to acquiring this book contract. I bask in gratitude for Michael's impact in my life. Michael, I am so blessed to be loved by you, wise owl.

I offer my deepest thanks to Haven Iverson who picked me out of a crowd and welcomed me into the family of Sounds True authors. Thank you for your detailed attention to making this book everything it could be. Thanks to Jennifer Brown, Jennifer Holder, Stephen Lessard, Kriste Peoples, Anastasia Pellouchoud, and, of course, Tami Simon, for your roles in this magical process of bringing this book to life.

Thanks to my literary agents, Laura Yorke and Carol Mann—and Linda Sivertson who connected us.

Thank you, Pam Liflander. I'm in awe of your powers and steeped in gratitude for your hand in building the Pleasure

Revolution. What a profound pleasure to be changing the world together with you.

Thank you, Marisa Clementi, for creating and cooking the sumptuous recipes that appear in this book. My animal purrs with extra pleasure when we are together in the kitchen.

I thank all my teachers, guides, friends, and helpers who have nurtured the seeds of wisdom inside me so that I can now share in this book. Thanks also to the many students and clients whose invitation to support them permitted me the opportunity to rise to the challenge and learn so much along the way.

There are so many others who have helped me in one vital way or another on the path to writing this book.

Gum Broomstick, who taught me to trust nature. Your rainforest abode will always be my spiritual home.

Starhawk, thank you for teaching me that pleasure is sacred, and for being a role model for honoring the earth and worshiping the divine feminine. What a thrill to have met you and to have built a herb spiral together.

Ilan "Apurva" Kafri, beloved dark shark, may I swim in the waters of your wisdom forever.

Joshua Rosenthal, our chance meeting in India changed the course of my destiny. Your school, the Institute for Integrative Nutrition, inspired me to move from the land of my birth, Australia, to the United States, and to the career that has led to this book being born. Thank you, Josho.

Bill Hedberg, thanks for introducing me to my animal. She and I are both eternally grateful for all the wisdom and healing you have shared with us.

Regena Thomashauer (a.k.a. "Mama Gena"), your teachings liberated my soul and I've never looked back. Thank you for writing the foreword to this book.

Marc David, my deepest thanks and respect to you, my mentor in the psychology of eating, who showed me the science that makes pleasurable weight loss not only a viable way to lose weight, but the only sane, sustainable way. Your teachings give my heart courage and make my soul soar. You told me years ago that we are midwives of the feminine approach; thank you for your support in this book's birth.

Annie Lalla, soul sister and my heart's protectress, thank you for sculpting me over the many years of our friendship. Your wisdom continues to guide me through the oceans of love.

Alex Ehrlich, thank you for your phenomenal belief in me, and for your undeniable role in putting Pleasurable Weight Loss on the map.

Abby Faust and Beth Brown, my fearless right hand women at Pleasurable Weight Loss who have supported me every step of the way, I owe you my eternal thanks. Thanks also to all the volunteers of the "Pleasure Posse" over the years, whose devoted service has enabled countless lives to be changed at my Pleasure Camps.

Bryan Franklin and Jennifer Russell, thank you for grooming me as a movement leader and for being such key players in my ecology.

The musical artist known as NIMITAE (a.k.a. Bryan Franklin), thank you for composing the Temple of Erotic Innocence and so many more soul-rendering tracks. I will dance in your oasis of sacred sound through all time.

Jeremy Johnson, you gave me life-changing advice and the blessing of your belief in me, thank you.

Neon, my original belly dance teacher. Your DVDs changed my life and birthed a passionate belly dancer. My animal and I thank you deeply.

Sera Solstice, my tribal fusion belly dance teacher, thank you for the immense access to pleasure I have learned through your dance.

Becca Krauss, thank you for your devoted care of my female animal throughout all these years. She smiles in gratitude at the mention of your name.

Javier Regueiro, for teaching me to love all sides of myself, light and dark.

Michel Madie, fellow devotee of the animal, thank you for the epiphanies that have changed my life.

Techa Beaumont, Misha Falzone, Amber Webster, Jo Hoy, Birgitte Phillipedes, Jenna Ritter, Jade Netanya Ullman, Antonia Levy, Meike Früchtelicht, Lora Garcia, Mike "Jazzy" Flaherty, Paul English, Naomi Rosenblatt, Pamela Davenport, Peter Cryle, and Rosie Delicious, you each had a life-changing role in my life and powerfully supported me toward becoming the woman who has now written this book. Thank you for all your care.

To the Ladies of the Mistress Mind: Stacey Morgenstern, LiYana Silver, Alexis "Ali Shanti" Neely, KC Baker, Jennifer Russell, Nisha Moodley, Wendy Yalom. You are my backbone, an eternal source of pleasure and delight, comfort, and wisdom. Thank you for the most profound sense of belonging I've ever known. You have cradled me throughout this entire process of conceiving and birthing this book.

To my interviewees: Andrea Albright, Cecily Miller, Michaela Boehm, Geoffrey Miller, Christopher Ryan, Alexandra Jamieson, Theresa Stevens, Tenley Wallace, Amber Hartnell, Annie Lalla, Renée Stephens, Gina Schatz, Sheri Winston, Ethan Depweg, Dara Cole, Alexis Neely, Aarona Pichinson, Pamela Morgan, Morgana Rae, Hemalayaa Behl, Cynthia Stadd, Amy Verebay, LiYana Silver, Tonya Leigh, Joshua Pellicer, Michel Madie, Theresa Stevens, Amber Lupton, Layla Martin, Ariel White, Saida Désilets, and Ilan Kafri.

To the extraordinary women in my life: Claire Cottone, Rose Cole, Sarah Jenks, Jess Johnson, Laura Hollick, Emily Rubin, Gabrielle Sundra, Laura Reid, Sonya Stewart, Kim Iglinsky, Julia Marayanska, Melanie Boylai, Kate Niebauer, Lisa Fabrega, Becca Fresco, Jules Cazedessus, Tbird Luv, Sophie Solomon, Kristen Domingue, Ruth Barron, Elie Calhoun, Kyra Reed, Lalita Salins, Lori Sutherland, Meggan Watterson, Liz Dialto, Jana Astanov, Alexis Sheppard, Shana James, Alia Hall, Erin Stutland, Gina DeVee, Kayce Neill, Eve Colantoni, Sabrina Chaw, Rachel Rofe, Alena Watters, Veena Sidhu, Julia Allison, Elizabeth Purvis, Emily Tepper, Heather Pierce, Bonnie Fahy, Sofiah Thom, Sacha Lalla, Katiyana Williams, Jenny Sauer-Klein, Julia Alison, Chelsea O'Brien, and Myvanwy Fleur, thank you all for being inspirational living embodiments of the Divine Feminine.

Theresa Stevens, exquisite embodiment of body joy, my animal is in ecstasy dancing with you. Thank you for your inspiration and wisdom.

Amber Otto, my favorite audience, your radiant heart ever opens me to deeper wisdom.

Layla Martin, Ariel White, and Saida Désilets, high priestesses of pleasures, my muses, my playmates, thank you for being my sacred accomplices in the Pleasure Revolution.

To the extraordinary men in my life: Eric Neuner, Warwick Saint, Nathan Patmor, Gregory Kellett, Stefan Pildes, Reid Mihalko, Philippe Lewis, Raj Sundra, Anant Jesse, Andrew Simpson, Robert Bienstock, David Hassell, Durian Songbird, John Taylor, Gio Cavalieri, Nat Mundell, Bear Kittay, Steve Bearman, David Niebauer, Guy Sengstock, John Seed, Sol Sebastian, Bryan Bayer, Vishen Lakhiani, Kerry Konrad, Shane Metcalf, Adam Gilad, Bodhi Seed, Christopher Ferrouge, Hitch McDermid, and Android Jones, thank you all for being inspirational living embodiments of the Divine Masculine.

Akil Davis, thank you for training my voice for recording the audio version of this book. The precious gifts you share with me offer endless joy and inspiration.

Marc Gafni, thank you for your songs, stories, wisdom, inspiration, and ceaseless support.

Cypher Zero (Sebastian Perluna), you liberated and empowered my animal in countless ways. Thank you, my journey with you was a priceless gift.

Mark Read, thank you for taking me under your wing in all the ways you do.

Michael Costuros, I give thanks for the blessing you are in my life and your influence, love, and care in my journey on Mother Earth.

Eben Pagan, thank you for changing my life on so many levels. My gratitude is undying.

Marie Forleo and Josh Pais, for mentoring me to trust my impulses like never before.

Danielle LaPorte, thanks for turning up the heat under my ass in our Firestarter Session, making a stand for this book to be born.

Geneen Roth, Marianne Williamson, Dr. Christiane Northrup, Barbara Marx Hubbard, Naomi Wolf, and Sera Beak, thanks for paving the way for this book with your groundbreaking feminine leadership. Beth Kenkel, for being my angel in a critical moment of the creation of this book. Thank you for sheltering me in your beautiful forest home for my writer's retreat. Jane Axamethy of the Bakehouse, for nourishing my body with healing, homemade food that allowed me to nourish others with my healing words, thank you.

Kerry Olditch, the violin-playing pixie who captured my heart and enflamed my soul before you left the world so young.

Thanks for profound inspiration from Mother India, Osho, Dolano, Yoga, the Sacred Clown, Rainbow Family, Radical Faeries, the Omega Institute, Burning Man, Camp Mystic, and Running Springs Ranch.

Patricia and Daniel Ellsberg, my mother and father in-love, thank you for bringing Michael into this world, and for your boundless love and support of me.

My sister Sally Geagea and brother David Gray; we will always be the three monkeys.

My deepest possible bow of gratitude goes to my parents, Mary Fitzpatrick and Peter Gray. Thank you for your unconditional love and your most sacred gift of all: life itself. Lastly, I offer thanks to our Mother Earth, the Great Mother of All.

Additional Resources

FEMININE LEADERSHIP

Alexis Neely is changing the way we make personal finance and relationship decisions with her Eyes Wide Open model of life and business: awake, aware, and on your terms. Visit eyeswideopenlife.com.

Amber Hartnell lives in service to revealing the wholeness and beauty at the heart of all she touches, a graceful guide in the process of dissolving fear and resistance to access the core and allow the intrinsically intelligent flow of love to in-form life. Visit amberhartnell.com.

Cecily Miller, PhD(c), has a private, therapeutic practice with pregnant women and couples around the world who are excited to be the parents they want to be and to evolve into the family their babies deserve. Visit letsbevolve.com.

Nisha Moodley is a women's leadership coach who believes that the world will be set free by women who are free, and that sisterhood is key to a woman's freedom. Visit nishamoodley.com.

Patricia Ellsberg is a social change activist, meditation teacher, and spiritual coach. In 1971, she helped her husband, Daniel Ellsberg, release to the press the Pentagon Papers, a top secret study of US involvement in Vietnam, which contributed to Nixon's resignation and an end to the Vietnam War. Visit patriciaellsberg.net.

Stacey Morgenstern is the cofounder of Holistic MBA, an international coach training school that creates leaders in the art, science, and business of transformation. Visit holisticmba.com.

SENSUALITY AND SEXUALITY EDUCATORS

Annie Lalla is a philosopher, thought leader, and love coach. Annie helps clients develop romantic esteem, resolve toxic patterns, diffuse conflict, assuage shame/blame, and cultivate deep, resilient relationships that last a lifetime. Visit annielalla.com.

Ariel White is an artist, entrepreneur, activist, embodied muse of the modern renaissance, and the founder of evoLover, an online platform for women's sensual and creative expression. Visit evolover.com.

Chris Ryan, PhD, is the coauthor of *Sex at Dawn: The Pre-Historic Origins of Modern Sexuality,* together with his wife, Cacilda Jethá, MD. Visit chrisryanphd.com.

Geoffrey Miller, PhD, is a psychology professor at the University of New Mexico and author of *The Mating Mind, Spent,* and the forthcoming *Mate.* He teaches evolutionary psychology and human sexuality. Visit thematinggrounds.com.

Layla Martin is an expert in how to have epic orgasms and mind-blowing sex. She is one of the rare people initiated into real Tantra. Visit laylamartin.com.

LiYana Silver is a teacher, coach, mentor, and author helping entrepreneurial women redefine success to honor their feminine hearts and bodies. Visit liyanasilver.com.

Michaela Boehm creates a dynamic, experiential teaching style that combines more than fifteen years of experience as a counselor with in-depth training in the yogic arts. She teaches artful intimacy and polarity with David Deida. Visit michaelaboehm.com.

Michel Madie, DVM, PhD, is a veterinarian, poet, humanist, astrologer, soul-boxing healer, tantra educator, dancer, photographer, and master chef who teaches that giving and receiving well requires us, and leads us, to start and end with self-love. Visit michelmadie.com.

Regena Thomashauer (a.k.a. "Mama Gena") is an icon, teacher, author, mother, and creatrix of The School of Womanly Arts who teaches women to use the power of pleasure to have their way with the world. Visit mamagenas.com.

Saida Désilets, PhD, is an author, researcher, and leading-edge global advocate for Women's Erotic Genius. Visit saidadesilets.com.

Sheri Winston, CNM, RN, LMT, is an author, wholistic sexuality teacher extraordinaire, and founder of the Center for the Intimate Arts, where she offers empowering and integral erotic education for everyone. Visit intimateartscenter.com.

PLEASURABLE MOVEMENT GUIDES

Aarona Pichinson is a yoga teacher known for her dynamic and thoughtful classes, epic global adventure retreats, and as the founder of Yoga Soundscape where exceptional musicians play live as she guides a rhythmically aligned yoga and movement class. Visit yogaofnourishment.com.

Amy Dawn Verebay is a teacher, performer, ritualist, yogini, and breathwork practitioner. Amy shares her talents to bring joy and empowerment to diverse populations. Visit amyverebay.com.

Andrea Albright has helped hundreds of thousands of women lose weight in a natural way and feel confident in bikinis. Visit mybikinibutt.com.

Bill Hedberg has dedicated his life to helping people come back to, make sense of, and mature themselves through the ritual of physical conditioning. Visit shentaostudio.com.

Dara Cole is the founder of Sacred, a groundbreaking movement studio in Brooklyn, NY. She is a master space-holder for healing the division between fitness and pleasure. Visit sacredbrooklyn.com.

Gina Schatz is a board-certified integrated bodywork therapist who believes it is possible to live in a world where people are pain free and is on a mission to make that a reality. Visit ginaschatz.com.

Hemalayaa is a leader in conscious movement who is transforming lives through Bollywood dance, Ayurveda, and yoga. Visit hemalayaa.com.

Neon is an acclaimed dancer, choreographer, dance fitness instructor, and the founder of World Dance New York—the world's largest producer of women's dance instruction, fitness, and lifestyle videos. Visit worlddancenewyork.com.

Tenley Wallace is a temple dancer, yogini, dakini, herstorian, and collector of dance and temple arts for the exploration and embodiment of the Sacred Feminine. Visit templetribalfusion.com.

Theresa Stevens is the author of *30 Days to Dance Your Way to BodyJoy: How to Get the Body & Beauty of Your Dreams with Pleasure, Joy & Dance*. She is a professional samba dancer and a pleasurable fitness coach, helping women all over the world feel sexy, beautiful, and energized through the pleasure of shaking their hips and booties. Visit shakeyourbootydance.com.

PLEASURABLE EATING COACHES

Alexandra Jamieson is a chef, coach, cravings whisperer, co-creator of the film *Super Size Me,* and author of the book *Women, Food, and Desire.* Visit alexandrajamieson.com.

Cynthia Stadd, EPC, is a pioneering practitioner and educator, leading women to permanently end their food and body war. Visit cynthiastadd.com.

Joshua Rosenthal, MScEd, is the founder and primary teacher of Integrative Nutrition who is committed to the simple idea that if we can change what people eat, we could help change the world. Visit integrativenutrition.com.

Marc David, MA, is the founder of the Institute for the Psychology of Eating, a leading visionary, teacher, nutritional psychology expert, and the author of the classic and bestselling books *Nourishing Wisdom* and *The Slow Down Diet.* Visit psychologyofeating.com.

Marisa Clementi, founder of Beauty in Every Bite, believes that food is love when we create meals that have been grown and prepared with care, that rest on a beautifully set table, and that leave the body satisfied, the mind at ease, and the soul in bliss. Visit beautyineverybite.com.

Pamela Morgan has been praised for her work as a caterer, culinary instructor, event planner, and cookbook author. She is the owner of the private event firm Flirting with Flavors. Visit flirtingwithflavors.com.

Renée Stephens, PhD, is dedicated to ending the weight struggle and enabling people around the world to share their souls' gifts. Visit reneemethod.com.

Tonya Leigh is a master-trained life coach, a former registered nurse, trained sommelier, and devout Francophile who inspires women to create lives of ease, elegance, and everyday ecstasy. Visit tonyaleigh.com.

PLEASURABLE STYLE COACH

Megan Chenoweth is a style coach who has the pleasure of lovingly guiding women to look, and thus feel, their best through the gift of style. Visit southernfemme.com.

SPIRITUAL TEACHER

Javier Regueiro works with Ayahuasca and San Pedro/Huachuma in Pisac, Peru, and is the author of the book *Ayahuasca: Soul Medicine of the Amazon Jungle.* Visit ayaruna.com.

About the Author

JENA LA FLAMME is a weight loss expert and the founder of the Pleasurable Weight Loss movement. Her profound teachings show that pleasurable weight loss is neither a contradiction nor an oxymoron. During her ten-year struggle with food, weight, and bad body image, Jena despised her body and was highly suspicious of pleasure. This lasted until she discovered that her issue wasn't that she was having too much pleasure, it was that she wasn't having enough! As she learned to trust the wisdom of her female body and to trust pleasure, she came to peace with food. Her figure and her body image transformed. Since then, Jena has devoted her life to showing women around the world how to be in tune with the innate wisdom of their bodies and how they, too, can be at peace with food while feeling great every step of the way. She takes a fierce stand for all women to take pride in themselves and their feminine nature.

Jena works with women of all ages through live Pleasure Camps, online programs, a popular website, social media outlets, and private coaching. Raised in Ireland and Australia, Jena now lives and teaches in New York City, but she prides herself on being a gypsy at heart.

Jena's unique approach to weight loss has made her a sought-after teacher. She has been featured in *Elle, Glamour,* and *Prevention* magazines. For more information, visit jenalaflamme.com.

About Sounds True

SOUNDS TRUE is a multimedia publisher whose mission is to inspire and support personal transformation and spiritual awakening. Founded in 1985 and located in Boulder, Colorado, we work with many of the leading spiritual teachers, thinkers, healers, and visionary artists of our time. We strive with every title to preserve the essential "living wisdom" of the author or artist. It is our goal to create products that not only provide information to a reader or listener, but that also embody the quality of a wisdom transmission.

For those seeking genuine transformation, Sounds True is your trusted partner. At SoundsTrue.com you will find a wealth of free resources to support your journey, including exclusive weekly audio interviews, free downloads, interactive learning tools, and other special savings on all our titles.

To learn more, please visit SoundsTrue.com/freegifts or call us toll-free at 800-333-9185.

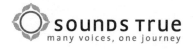

sounds true

many voices, one journey